Pharmacy and Medicine in Ancient Egypt

Pharmacy and Medicine in Ancient Egypt

Proceedings of the conference held in Barcelona (2018)

Edited by

Rosa Dinarès Solà
Mikel Fernàndez Georges
Maria Rosa Guasch-Jané

Archaeopress Egyptology 34

ARCHAEOPRESS PUBLISHING LTD
Summertown Pavilion
18-24 Middle Way
Summertown
Oxford OX2 7LG
www.archaeopress.com

ISBN 978-1-78969-770-4
ISBN 978-1-78969-771-1 (e-Pdf)

Cover: Sekhmet statues set up at Karnak during the reign of Amenhotep III (Dynasty 18), possibly as the focus of worship to terminate or avert plagues. Temple of Mut, Karnak. (Photograph courtesy of C. Price, The University of Manchester, December 2017).
Drawing of surgical instruments adapted from the Kom Ombo surgical instrument scene.

Contents

Preface and Acknowledgement

This monograph comprises the Proceedings of the Third International Conference on Pharmacy and Medicine in Ancient Egypt - EGYPHARMED 2018.

www.egypharmed2018.com

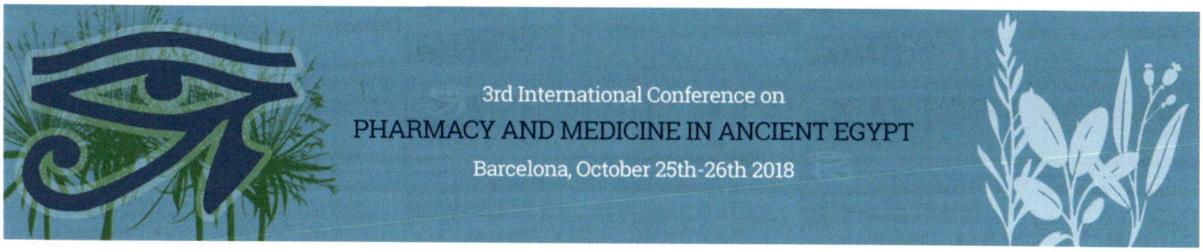

Following a first conference in Cairo (Egypt) in 2007 and a second in Manchester (UK) in 2008, on the 25th and 26th of October 2018, the Third International Conference on Pharmacy and Medicine in Ancient Egypt was held at Alimara Hotel in Barcelona (Catalonia).

The Organizing Committee

The team was formed by Dr. Rosa Dinarès Solà (Radiologist and Egyptologist), Dr. Mikel Fernandez Georges (Biologist, Egyptologist and Linguist) and Dr. Maria Rosa Guasch-Jané (Pharmacist and Egyptologist).

The Scientific Committee

Honorary President: Prof. Rosalie David, Emeritus Professor of Egyptology at The University of Manchester (UK).

President: Dr. Miguel Sánchez, Chief of Pathology and Medical Director of the Leslie Simon Breast Care and Cytodiagnosis Center at Englewood Hospital and Medical Center (USA).

Vice-president: Prof. Salima Ikram, Distinguished Professor of Egyptology at the American University in Cairo (Egypt) and Invited Professor at Yale University (USA).

Advisors:

Professor Eva-Maria Geigl, Co-director of the Epigenome and Paleogenome laboratory of the Institut Jacques Monod, University Paris-Diderot (Paris 7)/CNRS in Paris (France).

Dr. Albert Isidro, Consultant Orthopedist from Hospital Universitari Sagrat Cor in Barcelona and Aggregate Professor in Medicine at Universitat de Barcelona.

Dr. Jesús Herrerín López, PhD in Biological Sciences. Associate Professor of Biology at the Autonomous University of Madrid (Spain).

Professor Frank Rühli, Professor of Medicine at the University of Zurich (Switzerland) and Director of the Swiss Mummy Project.

Professor Lisa Sabbahy, Professor of Egyptology at the American University in Cairo (Egypt) and Program director of the MA in Egyptology and Coptology at AUC.

Dr. Sahar Saleem, Professor of Radiology at Kasr Al-Ainy, Faculty of Medicine of the Cairo University (Egypt) and Leading member of the Egyptian Mummy Project (Egypt).

The EGYPHARMED 2018 conference included presentations on new research and advances in the topics covered in the first two conferences.

The meeting displayed the most recent pharmaceutical and medical studies on human remains and organic and plant material from ancient Egypt, together with discussions on textual and iconographical evidence related to this subject in order to evaluate the knowledge and advances we have made on pharmacy, veterinary and human medicine in Ancient Egypt.

The Conference programme combined plenary sessions, oral communications and posters, and discussions which provided a forum to establish interdisciplinary collaborations between researchers and research groups that propose breakthrough studies on pharmacy, veterinary science and medicine in Ancient Egypt.

Participation in the conferences and posters ranged from distinguished researchers and professors from academic institutions, museums and universities, to postgraduates and doctoral students at the beginning of their careers.

The inaugural lecture was given by Professor Rosalie David, to whom we convey special thanks for her collaboration and participation.

The keynote lectures were by Professors Rosalie David (University of Manchester, UK), Salima Ikram (American University in Cairo, Egypt), Eva-Maria Geigl (Institut Jacques Monod in Paris, France), Frank Rühli (University of Zürich, Switzerland) and Sahar Saleem (Cairo University, Egypt).

Furthermore, special communications were presented by Professor Lisa Sabbahy (American University in Cairo, Egypt), Dr. Albert Isidro (University Hospital Sagrat Cor, Catalonia), Dr. Jesús Herrerín (Autonomous University of Madrid, Spain) and Dr. Rosa Dinarès Solà (General University Hospital of Catalonia).

The lectures and posters covered a wide range of topics and visions within this field of medicine.

We would specially like to thank the support and help of the following institutions:

- Associació Espanyola de Farmacèutics de la Indústria (AEFI)- secció catalana
- Col·legi de Farmacèutics de Barcelona
- Col·legi de Metges de Barcelona
- Institut Català d'Arqueologia Clàssica (ICAC)
- Museu Egipci de Barcelona
- Institut d'Estudis del Pròxim Orient Antic, Universitat Autònoma de Barcelona

Finally, we would like to especially thank Mr. Jordi Ruiz Camargo for his generous collaboration and to both Patricia Ruiz Villar and Patricia Rodriguez Corbera for the smooth running of the sessions during the congress.

Participants could also enjoy the Gala Dinner at Senyor Parellada restaurant and visits to the medieval hospital of La Santa Creu and Roman Barcelona. The latter was courtesy of Dr. Josep Maria Palet, director of the Catalan Institute of Classical Archaeology (ICAC).

With regard to the Proceedings, we would like to express our gratitude to the publisher, Archaeopress, and the financial support from Fundació Uriach 1838, in particular Mr. Javier Uriach Torelló, and Col·legi de Metges de Barcelona (COMB) for the main funding of this edition, as well as the Catalan Institute of Classical Archaeology (ICAC).

Barcelona, April 2020

Rosa Dinarès Solà, Mikel Fernandez Georges and Maria Rosa Guasch-Jané

Conference Programme

25 OCTOBER 2018 (Thursday)

9h-9:30h: Registration

9:30h-10h: Opening

Session chair: Professor Lisa Sabbahy, American University in Cairo (Egypt)

1st session: Medicine in Ancient Egypt

10-10:45h Keynote speaker: Professor Rosalie David, University of Manchester (UK)

'Epidemics and their aftermath in Ancient Egypt'

10:45h-11h: Coffee break

11h-13:30h: Communications

13:30-15h: Lunch

Session chair: Dr. Maria Rosa Guasch-Jané, director of the Wine of Ancient Egypt/ EGYWINE Project (Catalonia)

15-15:30h Keynote speaker: Professor Salima Ikram, American University in Cairo (Egypt)

'Images and analyses: Recent advances in mummy studies'

15:30-16h Special communication: Professor Lisa Sabbahy, American University in Cairo (Egypt)

'An update on our understanding of disease in Ancient Egypt'

Session chair: Professor Salima Ikram, American University in Cairo (Egypt)

2nd Session: Pharmacy and Vet in Ancient Egypt

16h-17:30h: Communications

17:30h-18h Keynote speaker: Professor Eva-Maria Geigl, Institut Jacques Monod, Paris (France)

'An Egyptian cat tale told by ancient DNA?'

26 OCTOBER 2018 (Friday)

Session chair: Professor Frank Rühli, University of Zürich (Switzerland)

9-9:45h Keynote speaker: Sahar Saleem, Cairo University (Egypt)

'Ancient Egyptian medicine and health in the eyes of modern science'

3rd Session: Palaeopathological diagnosis and New techniques applied to the study of human remains

9:45h-10:45h: Communications

10:45h-11h: Coffee break

Session chair: Professor Rosalie David, University of Manchester (UK)

11-11:30h Keynote speaker: Frank Rühli, University of Zürich (Switzerland)

'Biomedical research on ancient Egyptian mummies: General perspectives and latest findings in the Valley of the Kings (KV 31, KV 40, KV 64) and Sheikh Abd el-Qurna (TT95)'

11:30h-13:30h: Communications

13:30-15h: Lunch

Session chair: Dr. Mikel Fernández, University of Barcelona (Catalonia)

15:00-15:30h Special communication: Dr. Albert Isidro, University Hospital Sagrat Cor (Catalonia)

'Bone cancer in Ancient Egypt. State of Art'

4th session: Mummification and Variations

15:30h-17:00h: Communications

17-17:30h Special communication: Dr. Jesús Herrerín, Autonomous University of Madrid (Spain)

'New light on the mummification process: attempts to improve the body for the afterlife'.

17:30-18h Special communication: Dr. Rosa Dinarès Solà, University Hospital General of Catalonia (Catalonia)

'Ebers and Edwin Smith papyri compared to paleopathological data found in bones and mummified remains'.

18h-18:15h: Conclusions

Posters session: 1h

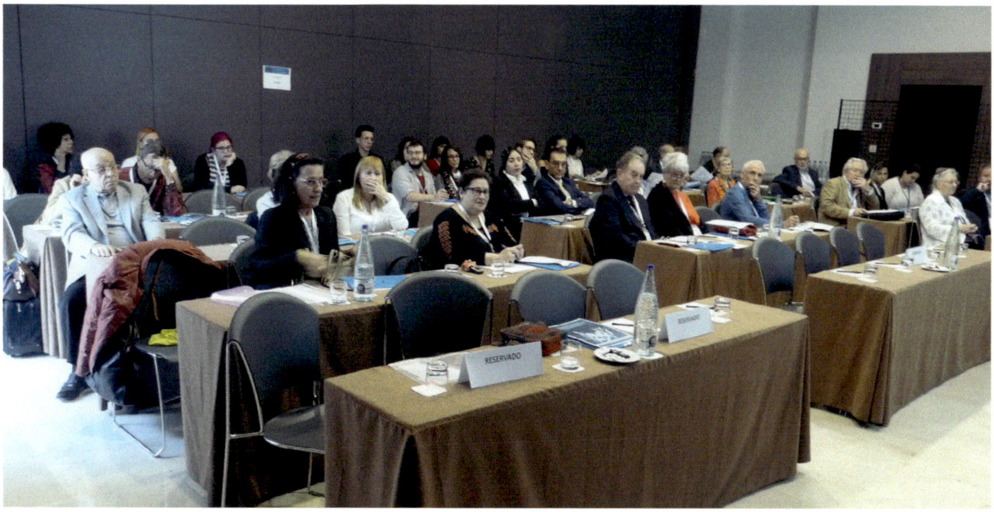

Third International Conference on Pharmacy and Medicine in Ancient Egypt (October 25-26, 2018)

Introduction

The main aims of this series of conferences are: first, to evaluate the knowledge and advances we have made relating to ancient Egyptian pharmacy, and veterinary and human medicine; and secondly, to provide an opportunity for researchers and research groups to establish interdisciplinary collaborations. The first conference was held at the National Research Centre, Cairo (March 19-22, 2007) and the second in Manchester (September 1-2, 2008); the meeting in Aswan, planned for 2012, did not materialise, and so the third conference was arranged for Barcelona.

The Barcelona conference was hosted by the Institut d'Estudis del Pròxim Orient Antic, Universitat Autònoma de Barcelona. It included some of the most recent pharmaceutical and medical studies on human remains and organic and plant materials from ancient Egypt, and focused on related textual and iconographic evidence, and the development and application of various biomedical/scientific techniques to identify evidence in ancient organic and inorganic remains.

Thirty papers (including three posters) were presented by authors from nine countries. The *Keynote Lectures* included: 'Epidemics and their aftermath in Ancient Egypt' (Professor Rosalie David, University of Manchester, UK); 'Images and analyses: recent advances in mummy studies' (Professor Salima Ikram, American University in Cairo, Egypt); 'An Egyptian cat tale told by ancient DNA?' (Professor Eva-Maria Geigl, Institut Jacques Monod, Paris, France); 'Ancient Egyptian medicine and health in the eyes of modern science' (Professor Sahar Saleem, Cairo University, Egypt); and 'Biomedical research on ancient Egyptian mummies: general perspectives and latest findings in the Valley of the Kings (KV 31, KV 40, KV64) and Sheikh abd el-Qurna' (Professor Frank Rühli, University of Zurich, Switzerland).

There were also four *Special Communications*: 'An update on our understanding of disease in ancient Egypt' (Professor Lisa Sabbahy, American University in Cairo, Egypt); 'Bone cancer in ancient Egypt: state of the art' (Dr Albert Isidro, University Hospital Cor, Catalonia); 'New light on the mummification process: attempts to improve the body for the afterlife' (Dr Jesús Herrerín, Autonomous University of Madrid, Spain); and 'Ebers and Edwin Smith Papyri compared to palaeopathological data found in bones and mummified remains' (Dr. Rosa Dinarès Solà, University Hospital General of Catalonia, Catalonia).

The conference papers discussed a wide range of material. This included: assessment of the current state of the subject area, including ethical approaches to human remains; analyses of the prescriptions, recipes and terms in the medical papyri; human medicine (pharaonic to Coptic periods, and comparisons with systems in neighbouring lands); medical personnel; veterinary medicine; and research methodology (including work in the field, experimental mummification, and some new approaches to medical imaging, palaeopathology, and aDNA identification).

Over the past five decades, a variety of conferences have addressed issues related to textual, archaeological and palaeopathological studies on mummies from different countries. Also, regular conferences have covered many aspects of Egyptology. Although papers on ancient Egyptian medicine and pharmacy have sometimes been presented at these events, this subject area has never been their main focus. This current series of conferences is unique in that it provides a specific forum where medicine and pharmacy can be discussed within the particular context of ancient Egypt.

Over the past century, it has been the custom to disseminate research in this field through academic journals (in numerous languages) which are dedicated to Egyptology, medicine, forensics, various sciences, technology, anthropology, history, archaeology, and museology. Given this wide range of publication, both the academic researcher and the general reader may sometimes find difficulty in accessing this material.

However, for this conference series, the papers are readily available: presented together in two monographs (in this publication, and in J. Cockitt and R. David (eds.) 2010. *Pharmacy and Medicine in Ancient Egypt: Proceedings of the conferences held in Cairo (2007) and Manchester (2008).* Oxford: Archaeopress). Now this pattern has been established, we hope that similar publications will continue to be a key feature of future meetings.

International academic interaction and co-operation are important in our subject area. Programmes arranged around venues in different countries also provide excellent opportunities for conference participants to visit local places of special interest. Tours in Barcelona included the Egyptian Museum, the Medieval Hospital of Santa Creu, and local Roman sites. The Gala Dinner (at the Senyor Parellada Restaurant) was another highlight of our time in this beautiful city.

The continuation of these conferences is vitally important for the continuation and development of this subject. Now well-established, it is hoped that similar programmes will continue on a regular basis in the future.

Rosalie David
The University of Manchester (UK)
Honorary President of the Scientific Committee
September 2019

Financial support for this edition provided by:

FUNDACIÓ URIACH 1838

Col·legi de Metges de Barcelona

and

ICAC Institut Català d'Arqueologia Clàssica

Clima FRED

EGY WINE

Antibacterial Analysis of the Minerals Used for Ocular Remedies in Ancient Egypt

Marc Argilés
marc.argiles@upc.edu
Department of Optics and Optometry,
Technical University of Catalonia

Roger Sabi
Maria Soledad Marqués-Calvo
Department of Optics and Optometry,
Technical University of Catalonia

Abstract: Ancient recipes for treating diseases are described in Ebers and Edwin Smith papyruses, which combine three types of ingredient of different origin: vegetal, animal and mineral. The aim of this study was to observe in vitro the efficacy of antibacterial properties for some of the minerals used to treat ocular pathologies in ancient Egypt. Two dilutions of the minerals chrysocolla, galena, lapis lazuli and malachite (1g in 5mL of distilled water, and 1g in 10 mL of distilled water) were used to investigate the effect of the concentration on two bacteria from the Spanish Type Culture Collection, Stapylococcus epidermidis (CECT 231) and Pseudomonas aeruginosa (CECT 110). Antimicrobial activity was determined by disc diffusion method plating 100 μL of each bacteria with a final concentration of 1×10^4 UFC/mL in duplicate and incubating at 37°C for 24 h. Bacterial inactivation depends on the microorganism and the mineral. Chrysocolla is the only mineral to decrease the population of both bacteria, while malachite is only effective against gram-positive bacteria (S.epidermidis). The study reveals a positive antimicrobial activity between some minerals used to treat ocular pathologies in ancient Egypt and the usual potential pathogenic bacteria that generate them.

Keywords: Egyptology; palaeopathology; ocular diseases; experiment

Introduction

A lot has been written about the ancient Egyptian papyruses to which we still have access, most of them about medical purposes. The study and analysis of these papyruses help us to learn more about ancient Egypt medical knowledge, specifically the pathologies and treatments used at that time. The presence of eye pathologies in ancient papyruses reveals a great knowledge of ocular structure, where the ambient conditions (sand and heat mostly) produced constant eye irritations and other eye pathologies. Within the large diversity of pathologies described in ancient papyruses we can find some specific to ocular and visual system. Ebers papyrus, dating approximately from 1534 BC (Güemez-Sandoval E, 2009), describes five different types of ocular injuries or pathologies: hemorrhages, opacities, inflammations, blindness and balls. Between these five groups we can distinguish about 13 different pathologies which were diagnosed thorough direct observation of the ocular structures. Treatments were based on three different substances: vegetal, animal and mineral, all mixed together. Regarding minerals, we can read in the literature about four different minerals used to make their recipes, (a) malachite, (b) chrysocolla, (c) lapis lazuli and (d) galena (Waterman R,1958 ; Nunn JF, 1996; Andersen S.Ry, 1997).

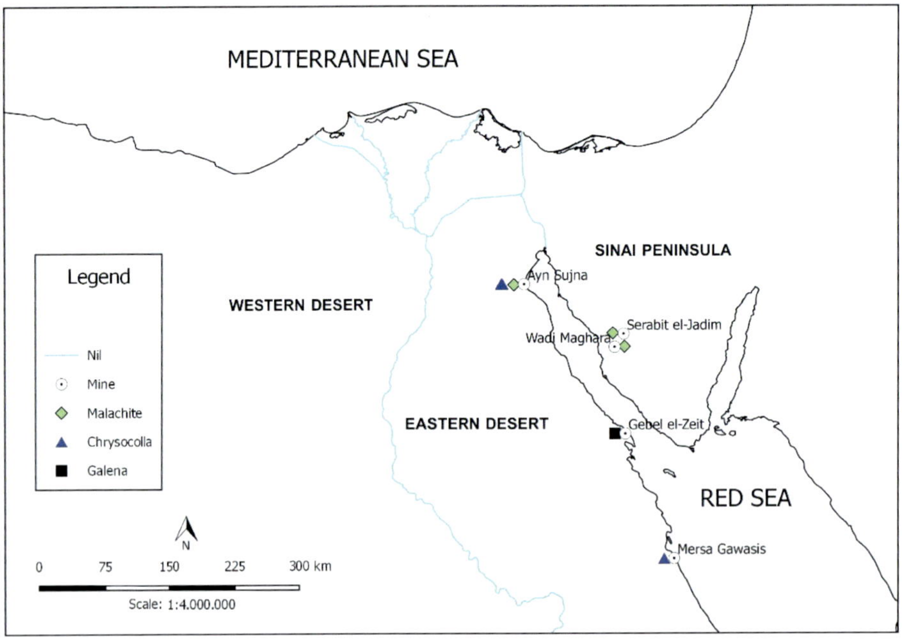

Figure 1. Mines and zones localization where ancient Egyptians probably obtained Malachite, Galena and Chrysocolla.

Copper-based minerals are malachite and chrysocolla. Malachite is a green copper carbonate hydroxide mineral, with the formula Cu2CO3(OH)2. Chrysocolla is a green hydrated copper phyllosilicate mineral with formula (Cu,Al)2H2Si2O5(OH)4·nH2O. Galena is principally lead-based, and lapis lazuli is not strictly a mineral, it is considered a semi-precious gemstone and is mostly azurite-based (giving the characteristic blue color). Note that the interpretation of these minerals is based on description of their color. For instance, green eye-paint described in Ebers 355,421 could be either malachite or chrysocolla. However, black eye-paint described in Ebers 430 and 367 has a high probability of referring to galena. We can find malachite, chrysocolla and galena in some mines and zones in ancient Egypt. Malachite in Wadi Maghara, Ayn Sujna and Serabit el-Jadim; Galena in Gebel el-Zeit; and Chrysocolla could be probably obtained in the region of Mersa Gawasis and Ayn Sujna (González-Tablas Nieto J, 2012). These mines and zones are situated in the Eastern Desert, near the Red Sea, and in the Sinai Peninsula (**Figure 1**). It is reasonable to think that the minerals were very common in this zone. Probably galena could also be obtained through trade. However, lapis lazuli was not naturally found in ancient Egypt and could only be obtained through trade, via the Silk Road. Some researchers claim that most of the lapis lazuli found in Egypt comes from a region located in the mountains of the Hindu Kush, named Badajshán, in present day Afghanistan (Del Cerro Linares C, 2011). Another possible use for these minerals is in the manufacture of kohl, the eye-liner used for cosmetic and magic purposes. The black and green colored paint was composed with galena and malachite (or chrysocolla).

In order to study the possible effectiveness of the treatments presented in ancient Egyptian recipes, we aim to analyze the possible antibacterial properties of pure malachite, chrysocolla, galena and lapis lazuli against the most common gram-positive and gram-negative bacteria.

Materials and methods

Published studies and databases of the mines were used for the previous microbiological analysis (Lefebure G, 1956). For this study, fine powder of galena, malachite, laurent and chrysocolla was obtained. Two dilutions of the minerals (1: 1g in 5mL of distilled water, and 2: 1g in 10 mL of distilled water) were used to investigate the effect of the concentration on the bacteria. Standard gram-positive and gram-negative bacteria strains for antibiotic testing, *Staphylococcus epidermidis* (CECT 231) and *Pseudomonas aeruginosa* (CECT 110) respectively, were used at a final concentration of 1 x 10^4 CFU/mL. Antimicrobial activity was determined by disc diffusion method, plating 100 µL of each bacteria in duplicate and incubating at 37°C for 24 h. One gram of each powder mineral was carefully placed on the culture media as a control (C). Image J program was used to determine the diameter of the inhibition rings.

Results

Results of the antimicrobial activity of both concentrations of the minerals are summarized in **Table 1**. The results show the extent of bacterial inactivity depending on the microorganism and the mineral. In this way, the effect of the concentration can be observed and, if the mineral has antimicrobial activity, the higher its intensity, the higher the concentration. Chrysocolla is the only mineral able to decrease the population of both bacteria, while malachite is only effective against gram-positive bacteria (*S.epidermidis*) (**Figure 2**).

Table 1. Antibacterial activity of the minerals on *S. epidermidis* (CECT 231) and *P. aeruginosa* (CECT 110) populations. Measure in mm.

	S. epidermidis			*P. aeruginosa*		
	1 (1 gr in 5 mL)	*2 (1 gr in 10 mL)*	*Control (1 gr)*	*1 (1 gr in 5 mL)*	*2 (1 gr in 10 mL)*	*Control (1 gr)*
Crysocolla	**9.0**	**6.0**	**16.0**	**11.0**	**10.0**	**24.0**
Galena	*0.0*	*0.0*	*0.0*	*0.0*	*0.0*	*0.0*
Lapislazuli	*0.0*	*0.0*	*0.0*	*0.0*	*0.0*	*0.0*
Malachite	**15.0**	**9.0**	**21.0**	*0.0*	*0.0*	*0.0*

Discussion

In this study we analyzed the efficacy of antibacterial properties for some of the minerals used to treat ocular pathologies in ancient Egypt. The minerals were selected based on the literature which demonstrates their use in the ancient papyri (Waterman R, 1958; Nunn JF, 1996; Andersen S.Ry, 1997). The geographical extraction of each mineral and the relationship with their use for remedies is relevant. Lapis lazuli is the only mineral that could not be extracted directly by the ancient Egyptians because it was not naturally found in deserts or mountains near the Nile or in the Red Sea. The only way to obtain this mineral was through trade. Galena, malachite and chrysocolla could be extracted through expeditions organized in the different mines and zones

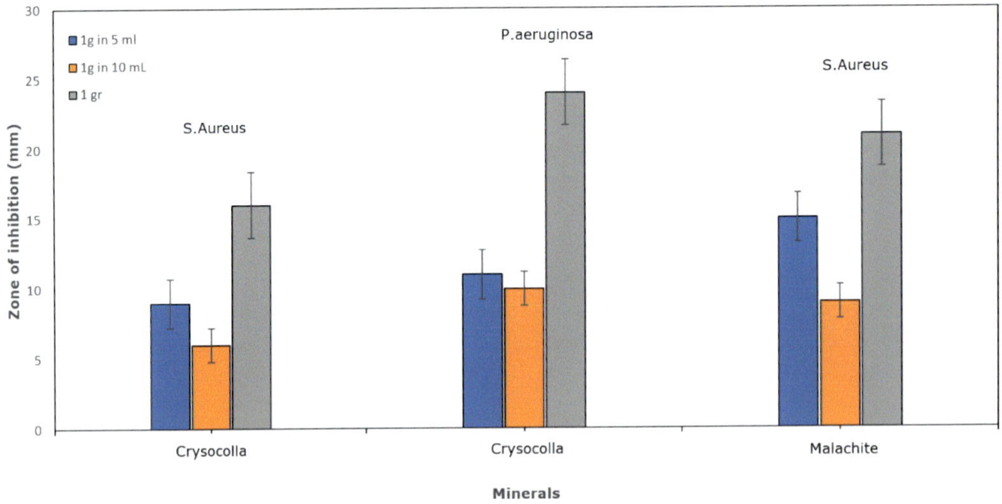

Figure 2. Zone of inhibition for the minerals Chrysocolla and Malachite. We plotted the positive results of the minerals in *S. epidermidis* and *P. aeruginosa*.

such as Ayn Sujna, Gebel el-Zeit, Mersa Gawasis, Serabit el-Jadim and Wadi Maghara (González-Tablas Nieto J, 2012).

Some studies shows that copper-based minerals could have antibacterial properties (Top A, Ülkü S, 2004;Williams LB, Haydel SE; 2010). Although in this study we try to replicate only the antibacterial properties of the minerals, we know that the ancient Egyptian recipes were made with different substances mixed together. For instance, we can read in Eber line 378 that the treatment for ocular inflammation was the use of lapis lazuli, crocodile dung and a magical spell, or in Ebers line 421 that the treatment for ectropion (an outward turning of the eyelid margin) a mix of chrysocolla, terebinth resin and ochre. We can discuss the real benefit of these treatments, but it is very interesting how the different and various remedies for distinct pathologies were used, which leads us to think about the advanced medicine they had in the past, based in observation, diagnosis and treatment. In this study we observed positive antibacterial properties for chrysocolla and malachite, copper-based minerals widely used for ancient eye make-up and ocular remedies. Moreover, the color of these minerals is important, for green (malachite and chrysocolla) meant health, and the black color (galena) represented death and the afterlife to the ancient Egyptians (Pinch G, 2004). Blue (from lapis lazuli) was associated with fertility and rebirth. We can barely think that ancient physicists knew about these antibacterial properties, but the possible real effect against eye infections due to these minerals is surprising. Also, it is interesting to note that ancient Egypt medicine was also based on magic and religious belief, since they believed that most of the diseases were caused by a curse (Campbell J, 2007). Nevertheless, the possible real antibacterial properties for the minerals described in this study raises the prospect of the rational treatment of disease and advanced medicine.

Conclusions

The study reveals a positive antimicrobial activity between some minerals used to treat ocular pathologies in ancient Egypt and the usual bacteria that generate them. Specifically, only those which are copper-based are effective. There is a possibility that Egyptian physicists recognized this efficacy empirically. Although we know the strong belief in magic and religion, the data reported here appear to support the assumption that these minerals described in the ancient papyruses have some positive effect against potential pathogenic bacteria. More accurate analysis with the pour plate method has to be conducted in order to quantify the antibacterial properties of these minerals.

References

Andersen, SRy 1997, *'The eye and its diseases in Ancient Egypt'. Acta Ophthalmologica Scandinavica,* vol.75, pp.338-344.

Campbell, J 2007, *Pharaohs and the first prescriptions. Pharmaceutical,* vol.279, pp.735–737.

Chatterjee, AK and Chakraborty, R and Basu, T 2014. 'Mechanism of antibacterial activity of copper nanoparticles', *Nanotechnology*, vol.*25*, no.13,135101.

David, R 2008, *'The art of healing in ancient Egypt: a scientific reappraisal'.* The Lancet, vol.372, pp.1802-1803.

Del Cerro Linares, C 2011, 'Azul para los dioses. De oriente a occidente: La búsqueda del Lapislázuli durante el III milenio A.C', *Revista sobre Oriente Próximo y Egipto en la antigüedad,* vol.13, pp.71-103.

González-Tablas Nieto, J 2012, *'La explotación egipcia de los recursos fuera del Valle del Nilo a finales de la Dinastía XII (C. 1870-1773 A. C.): Nubia, Asia y los desiertos'.* Unpublished thesis. Universidad de Salamanca.

Güemez-Sandoval, E 2009, 'El papiro Ebers y la oftalmología'. *Medigraphic artemisa en linea, Rev. Mex Oftalmol,* vol.83, no.2, pp.123-125.

Lefebure, G 1956, *'Essai sur la médicine égyptienne de l'époque pharaonique'.* Presses Universitaire de France. Paris.

Nunn, JF 1996, *Ancient Egypt Medicine.* ed British Museum Press. London.

Pinch, G 2004, *Egyptian mythology: A guide to the gods, goddesses, and traditions of ancient Egypt.* Oxford University Press, New York.

Raffi, M and Mehrwan, S and Bhatti, TM and Akhter, JI and Hameed, A and Yawar, W and ul Hasan MM 2010. 'Investigations into the antibacterial behavior of copper nanoparticles against Escherichia coli'. *Annals of microbiology,* vol. 60, no.1, pp.75-80.

Top, A and Ülkü, S 2004. 'Silver, zinc, and copper exchange in a Na-clinoptilolite and resulting effect on antibacterial activity'. *Applied Clay Science,* vol. 27, no.1-2, pp. 13-19.

Waterman, R 1958, *'Die altägyptischen Augenärzte'. Sudhoff's Archive fur Geschinchte di Medizin* , vol.42, pp.117-141.

Williams, LB and Haydel, SE 2010, 'Evaluation of the medicinal use of clay minerals as antibacterial agents'. *International geology review* , vol.52, no. 7-8, pp.745-770.

Epidemics and Their Aftermath in Ancient Egypt

Rosalie David

rosalie.david@manchester.ac.uk
Centre for Biomedical Egyptology, University of Manchester

Abstract: Ancient Egypt - a great politico-military power – had frequent contact with neighbouring lands. Opportunities for transmission of epidemic or pandemic diseases arose from population transfers (the result of incursions, military campaigns, prisoners-of-war, migrations and foreign settlements), climate and environmental conditions, cramped domestic arrangements, and intermittent famines. However, conclusive evidence of widespread plagues is lacking in Egypt: is this a false assumption, based on chance discovery and source limitations, or was the population too small to support the emergence of major epidemics? This paper examines the available evidence, and suggests that new immunological and molecular data should be sought.

Keywords: Egyptology; epidemics/plagues; disease; mummies (Egypt); palaeopathology

Introduction

As a great politico-military power, ancient Egypt was the centre of various cultural crossroads which ensured continuing contact with neighbouring lands. Population transfers – through incursions, military campaigns, prisoners-of-war, migrations and foreign settlements – also occurred, bringing Egypt into contact with Nubia, Asia Minor and the lands around the Mediterranean.

A two-way exchange of influences existed between Egypt and these regions: these included the transmission of disease, and of medical concepts and treatments (David 2017: 271-285).

Methods of transmitting medical skills and systems

Skills of Egyptian doctors

The medical skills of Egyptian doctors were internationally acknowledged. Documentary evidence includes a letter from the ruler of Ugarit to the Egyptian pharaoh requesting that he sends a doctor (Amarna archive EA 49) (Moran 1992); also, a Hittite king invited Egyptian doctors to his court (Geller 2010: 51), and later they held high positions at the Persian court.

Transmission between Egyptian and other medical systems

Transmission of medical knowledge also arose because foreigners sought cures at Egyptian temples, renowned as centres of healing. Other medical systems also had an impact on Egyptian treatments. For example, there are references to diseases and treatments of foreign origin in the Egyptian medical papyri (Leitz 2000) (e.g, a foreign incantation written in the Cretan language against the 'Canaanite illness' (London Medical Papyrus, Dynasty 18)). A letter from the Amarna archive (23) relates that the Mitannian king Tushratta sent a healing statue of the goddess Ishtar to the Egyptian court, perhaps in an attempt to alleviate the ill-health suffered

PHARMACY AND MEDICINE IN ANCIENT EGYPT
(ARCHAEOPRESS 2021): 6–14

by Amenhotep III. Later, migrations to Egypt during the Graeco-Roman Period brought Greek medicine into the country.

Sources of evidence for epidemic and pandemic diseases in Egypt and neighbouring lands

One might expect that continuing contact between Egypt and neighbouring lands would result in disease transmission. The unique climatic and environmental factors, religious beliefs and burial customs found in Egypt have ensured that a wealth of material has survived. This includes archaeological assemblages, textual records, and preserved human remains – all possible sources of evidence relating to epidemic and pandemic diseases.

Archaeological evidence of bodies disposed of during epidemics includes the finds at Tell el-Daba'a (Dynasty 13) and at the burial complex of Harwa and Akhimenru in western Thebes. The Amarna archive includes references to plagues. One mentions the disease that ravaged the Egyptian base at Sumar; in another (EA35), the king of Alashiya (Cyprus) tells the Egyptian king that he has only sent a small amount of copper to Egypt because all his copper-workers have been killed by a plague.

Contemporary references in non-Egyptian literature include the plague-prayers of the Hittite ruler, Mursil II. These describe an epidemic in Khatti that killed the kings Suppiluliumas and Arnuwanda II. Apparently transmitted by Egyptian soldiers taken prisoner at the battle of Amka in Syria in Dynasty 18, the disease continued to have an impact on the Hittites for twenty years.

Plagues and Epidemics in Egypt

Biblical Plagues

The best-known reference to an epidemic in Egypt occurs in the Bible (Marr and Malloy 1996:7-24). The description of the sixth plague (Exodus 9: 8-12) includes a festering skin condition (perhaps a symptom of an epidemic disease) that affected the Egyptians and their livestock. This may have been transmitted to humans from the livestock disease that characterised the fifth plague (Hoyte 1993: 285-286).

The tenth plague (Exodus 11: 1-12; 36), the death of the firstborn, may have been caused by toxins present in the morning meal, perhaps resulting from overnight pollution caused by locusts or black mould.

There has been considerable debate about this account (Hoffmeier 1996): was it allegorical; a memory-compilation of disconnected natural disasters; or an actual chain of events, perhaps even the first extant record of bubonic plague?

Bubonic Plague

It has been generally assumed that bubonic plague (*Yersinia pestis*) did not exist in pharaonic times, and currently there is only scanty, controversial evidence to contradict this (Davis *et al.* 1975: 147-173; Kozloff 2006: 36-46). There is no direct allusion to the disease in the medical papyri, although mention of the 'Tumours of Khons' may refer to the enlarged lymph glands (buboes) characteristic of bubonic plague (Nunn 1996: 95). The 'coal-black spots' (Hearst

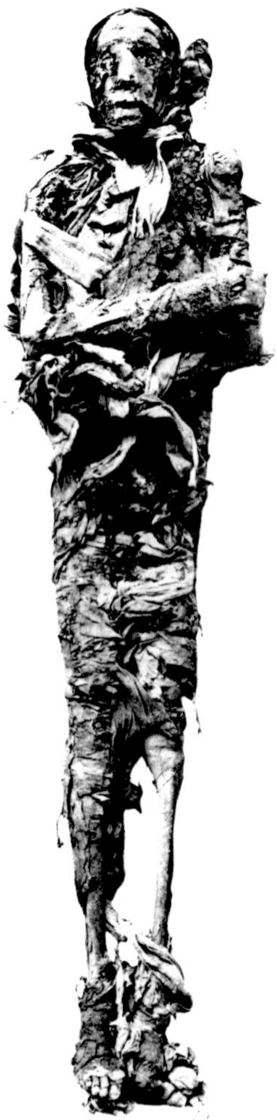

Siptah **Figure 1** The mummy of Pharaoh Siptah (Dynasty 19) showing a shortening of the left leg and gross deformity of the ankle. Cairo Museum.
(Photograph from G E Smith, *The Royal Mummies* (1912), pl. LXII, Fig. 1. Courtesy of the KNH Centre Archive, The University of Manchester).
Image 3.tif

Medical Papyrus H XI 12-15) and 'blood-red urine' (London Medical Papyrus 15: 8-10) may also refer to symptoms of this disease.

Rats and fleas play a crucial part in transmitting the causative bacillus for bubonic plague to a human population. The disease may have originated with the black rat (*Rattus rattus*), probably in northern India. However, recent Egyptian evidence may indicate a different scenario: that the disease was first associated with the Nile rat (*Arvicanthis niloticus*) whose flea then jumped to the black rat which had been accidentally imported into Egypt.

Remnants of the Nile rat have been discovered at Tell el-Daba'a (Dynasty 13). Emergency burials without funerary assemblages also occur here, perhaps indicating abandonment because of an epidemic, although no firm evidence of this has been found (Bietak 1996).

Remnants of human and animal fleas have been found at Tell el-Amarna (Dynasty 18) (Panagiotakopulu 2004: 269-275). The skeletal remains of labourers discovered in a cemetery there indicate an unusually low age-at-death (seven to twenty-five years). It is possible that they were victims of an epidemic, perhaps because their immune responses were compromised due to particularly arduous working conditions (Dabbs *et al.* 2015: 43-52).

Unsurprisingly, palaeopathological evidence of this disease is lacking: major symptoms of bubonic plague – high fever, tachycardia, headache and chills – would leave no trace on the body. Based on the evidence of a lung lesion, the pneumonic version of the disease has been tentatively identified in only one mummy (Ptolemaic Period).

However, the successful application of genetic techniques to identify plague in other ancient societies may yet produce encouraging results in Egyptian material (Drancourt and Raoult 2002: 105-109).

Malaria

This seasonal infection, caused by parasites of the genus *Plasmodium*, is usually transmitted to humans through the bite of an infected mosquito. The appropriate climatic and environmental conditions were present in the Fayoum (and possibly the Delta) in pharaonic and Graeco-Roman times. However, a lack of evidence initially led some researchers to conclude that malaria did not exist in ancient Egypt. There is no reference to the characteristic fever in the medical papyri, and the disease would not produce gross pathological changes in the human remains.

However, the *Para*Sight™-F test, an immunological tool developed to detect the antigen produced by *Plasmodium falciparum* in modern populations, has been adapted for ancient human remains (Miller *et al.* 1994: 31-32). In one study, the relevant antigen was successfully identified in seven out of eighteen samples taken from bodies spanning the Predynastic Period (*c.* 3000 BCE) to the Nubian Ballana Period (CE 350-550). Genetic techniques have also made a contribution (Sallares *et al.* 2000), including the tentative identification of *Plasmodium falciparum* in liver samples from mummies in the Dakhla Oasis (Rutherford 2008: 116-132).

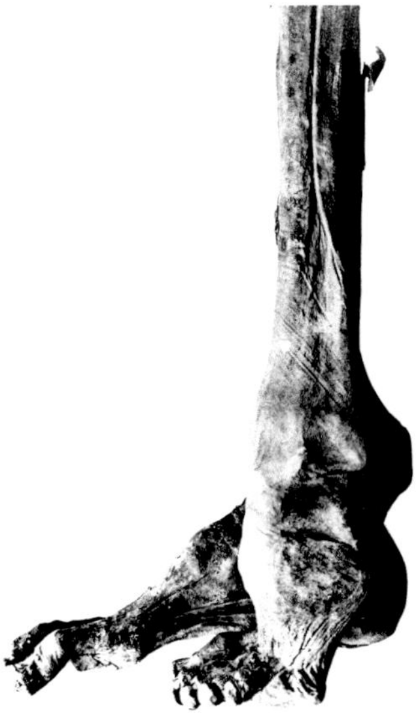

Figure 2 The deformity in the left leg and foot of Pharaoh Siptah (Dynasty 19) was originally identified as congenital clubfoot (talipes equino-varus). Radiological evidence indicates a neuromuscular disease, perhaps poliomyelitis. Cairo Museum. (Photograph from G E Smith, *The Royal Mummies* (1912), pl. LXII, Fig. 2. Courtesy of the KNH Centre Archive, The University of Manchester).

Poliomyelitis

When Grafton Elliot Smith unwrapped the mummy of King Siptah (Dynasty 19) in 1907 (Smith 1912), he noted a shortening of the left leg and a gross deformity of the ankle which he identified as congenital clubfoot (*talipes equino-varus*) (Figure 1). However, radiological studies suggest that it may be a neuromuscular disease, perhaps poliomyelitis (Dzierzykray-Rogalski and Prominska 1994) (Figure 2).

Other potential evidence for this disease in Egypt is rare (Mitchell 1900: 414-415). Unilateral shortening of the femur in a mummy from Deshasha (*c.* 700 BCE) may have resulted from poliomyelitis. A depiction of Roma, a temple door-keeper, on his funerary stela (Dynasty 18/19) shows him with a severely wasted and shortened leg; this may indicate clubfoot or poliomyelitis.

Even if these individual cases could be confirmed, there are no other identified cases. Since poliomyelitis does not occur in isolation, evidence to support any widespread occurrence of this disease in ancient Egypt is lacking.

Smallpox

When Grafton Elliot Smith unwrapped the mummy of King Ramesses V in 1905 (Smith 1912), the cutaneous vesicles on the face, neck, chest and lower abdomen were tentatively identified as smallpox (Figure 3). Electron microscopy and a radioimmunoassay were used to test this diagnosis in 1971, with inconclusive results. However, an immunoprecipitation test has since confirmed smallpox.

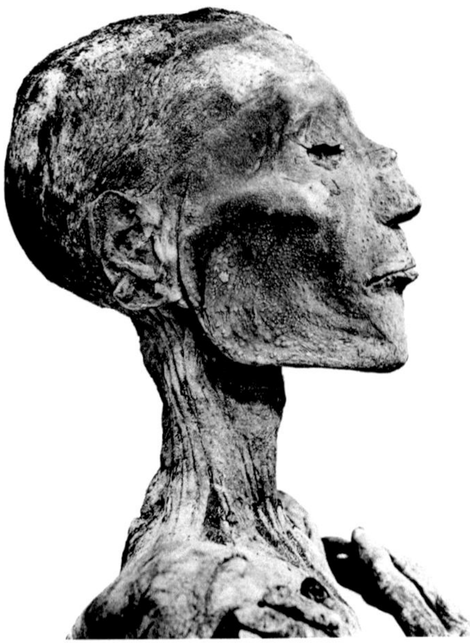

Figure 3 The mummy of Pharaoh Ramesses V (Dynasty 20). Immunological tests have confirmed the original tentative diagnosis of smallpox, based on cutaneous vesicles on the face (seen here) and other parts of the body. (Photograph from G E Smith, *The Royal Mummies* (1912), pl. LVI. Courtesy of the KNH Centre Archive, The University of Manchester).

There has been one other tentative diagnosis of smallpox, based on a skin lesion in another mummy (Dynasty 20) (Ruffer and Ferguson 1911: 1-3). However, smallpox has not been identified in other human remains, and the characteristic vesicles are not described in the medical papyri. There is no evidence that smallpox was ever widespread in Egypt (Hopkins 1980: 220); it is a density-dependent disease, and the population may have been too small to enable it to reach epidemic proportions (Strouhal 1996: 315-319).

Leprosy

There is no palaeopathological evidence of nodular leprosy in mummified remains from pharaonic times, possibly because these individuals were separated from society and had no access to mummification. In two passages in the Ebers Papyrus (874 and 877), one translator (Ebbell 1937) has interpreted the 'Tumours of Khons' as leprosy but other suggestions include cancer or bubonic plague.

Leprosy is confirmed in some examples from later periods (Møller-Christensen and Hughes 1996: 242-243): two skulls from Dakhla Oasis (*c.* 200 BCE); other skulls from sites near Aswan (fourth – seventh centuries CE); and in a mummy from a Coptic burial at Biga (sixth century CE).

Possible indications of leprosy were observed in the nasal area of the maxilla of Mummy 1770, unwrapped at the University of Manchester in 1975. It is hoped to re-examine this mummy, utilising new techniques to obtain more conclusive results.

Salmonella, Typhus and Typhoid

Hot weather and unsanitary water supplies undoubtedly encouraged the spread of these diseases, caused by contaminated food, water and milk. However, these acute illnesses would have resulted either in the patient's rapid demise or complete recovery, and would have left no trace on the body. The medical papyri refer to generic fevers but it is impossible to identify these with particular diseases.

The 'Asiatic' or 'Canaanite' Disease

Eight spells in the Edwin Smith Papyrus are the main literary source for this disease. These were intended to exorcise an annual epidemic in Egypt known as 'the pest of the year'

(Goedicke 1984: 91-105). Epidemics were thought to be brought by malignant deities, demons, the disembodied dead and the wind. The spells requested benign deities and spirits to protect and heal the afflicted, and to placate Sekhmet, the lioness-headed deity who brought disease (Figure 4). They identified breath, the arrows of night-demons (transporting Sekhmet's rage), and the wind as carriers of disease (this is the first extant reference to the concept that pestilence was windborne).

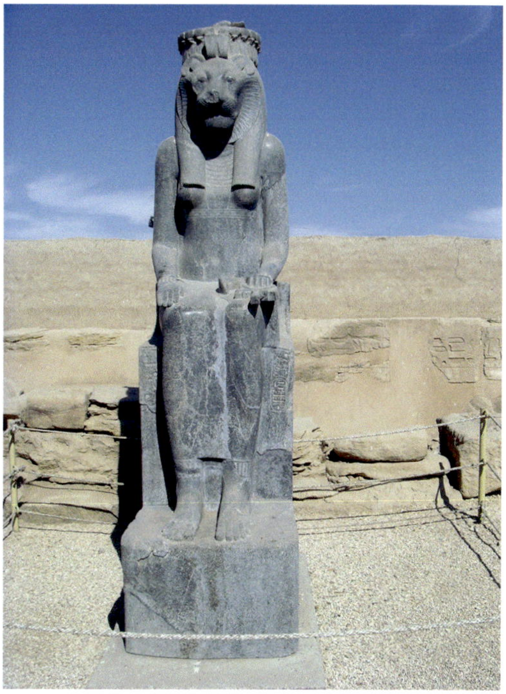

Figure 4 Statue of the lioness-headed goddess Sekhmet, regarded as the bringer of plagues and epidemics to Egypt. In an attempt to placate her and avert these disasters, she was worshipped as the principal deity of medicine. Dynasty 18. Temple of Mut, Karnak. (Photograph courtesy of K. White, The University of Manchester, December 2017).

The term 'Asiatic' may indicate that the disease originated outside Egypt, or perhaps inside a foreign enclave within Egypt, such as Tell el-Daba'a. Its arrival seems to have coincided with the Nile inundation, a time of general spiritual chaos and confusion. According to inscriptional sources, the disease was characteristically spread by air or breath, and accompanied by a fever that caused physical weakness; although it occurred regularly, it was not always fatal (Figure 5).

Since no specific symptoms are recorded, the disease cannot be clearly identified. Various suggestions, including Biblical plagues, malaria, typhoid and dengue fever, have been made; the most likely is that the 'pestilence of the year' embraced a diverse group of infectious diseases (Győry 2010: 81-84).

The Cyprian Plague

This plague carries the name of Cyprian, Bishop of Carthage (Tunisia), whose account describes the symptoms of the disease. It probably describes a series of epidemics that occurred in the third century CE, and decimated the Roman Empire.

Archaeological evidence from a funerary complex in western Thebes may link Egypt with these epidemics (Tiradritti 2014: 15-18). Originally the burial place of Harwa (TT37) and Akhimenru (TT404), the complex was subsequently used at least once for the disposal of a large number of corpses during a disease outbreak, possibly smallpox or measles.

Evidence included the remains of a large bonfire containing corpses, partially burnt bricks and pottery vessels that can be dated to the period (251 – 271 CE) of the Cyprian epidemics in the Roman Empire.

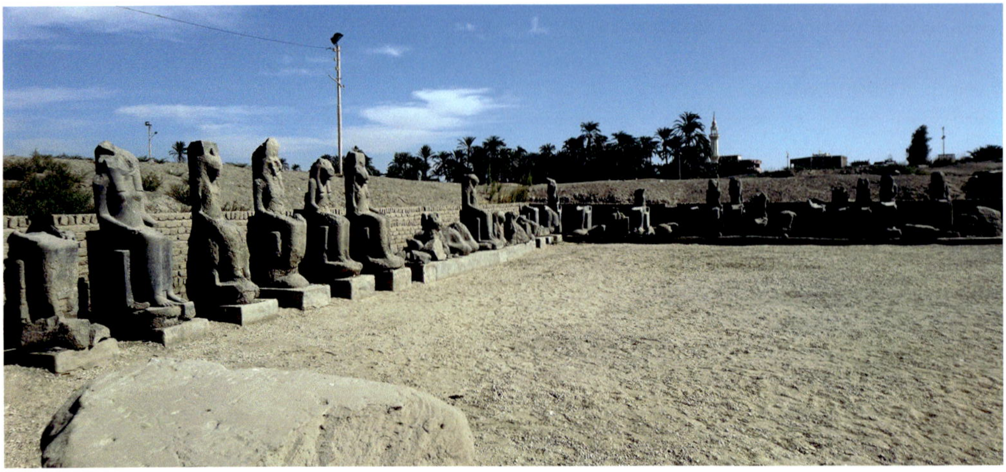

Figure 5 Large numbers of Sekhmet statues were set up at Karnak during the reign of Amenhotep III (Dynasty 18), possibly as the focus of worship to terminate or avert plagues. Temple of Mut, Karnak. (Photograph courtesy of C. Price, The University of Manchester, December 2017).

Conditions conducive to the spread, severity and aftermath of epidemics in Egypt and neighbouring areas

Several factors existed which could have promoted epidemic and pandemic diseases in Egypt and the surrounding lands. These included climatic and environmental conditions, cramped domestic accommodation, intermittent famines (which may have increased vulnerability to disease), and population movements that offered considerable opportunities for disease transmission.

However, there is no archaeological, textual or palaeopathological evidence of widespread, devastating plagues in Egypt (Sandison 1972: 213-224). This may be an inaccurate perception, influenced by the chance of discovery or limitations of the evidence.

Unlike the Classical accounts of epidemics in Greek and Roman times, there is no similar extant account from Egyptian sources. The medical papyri offer no identifiable description of epidemic symptoms. Formal historical texts (which focused on praising the king's achievements and his relationship with the gods) make no reference to plagues, although some sources (e.g., the Pessimistic Literature) may preserve a folk memory of appalling conditions associated with such events.

Relatively few human remains have been investigated, and these have mainly focused on the bodies of the elite, producing a generally unbalanced overview of disease patterns. Also, many indicators of epidemic disease are not preserved in human remains, or are difficult to detect with some diagnostic methods currently available.

Conclusion

The extent of epidemic disease and its role in pharaonic and Graeco-Roman times remains unclear. In order to answer some major questions, significant new data should be sought.

New insight could be provided by a reassessment of some of the medical papyri. An extensive examination of human remains is required, with a focus on immunological and molecular techniques which, despite their technical challenges, offer considerable opportunities.

However, although Egyptian and other texts suggest that widespread disease did occur, the conclusion may ultimately be reached that the population of pharaonic Egypt was perhaps too small to support the emergence of major epidemics.

Bibliography

Bietak, M. 1996. *Avaris. The Capital of the Hyksos. Recent Excavations at Tell el-Daba'a.* London: British Museum Press.

Dabbs, G. R., J. C. Rose, and M. Zabecki. 2015. The bioarchaeology of Akhetaten: unexpected results from a capital city, in S. Ikram, J. Kaiser and R. Walker (eds.) *Egyptian Bioarchaeology: humans, animals and the environment:* 43-52. Leiden: Sidestone Press.

David, R. 2017. Illness from afar: epidemics and their aftermath, in P. P. Creasman and R. H. Wilkinson (eds.) *Pharaoh's Land and Beyond: Ancient Egypt and Its Neighbours*: 211-285. Oxford: Oxford University Press.

Davis, D. H. S., A. F. Hallett and M. Isaacson. 1975. Plague, in W. T. Hubbert, W. M. McCulloch and P. R. Schnurrenberger (eds.) *Diseases Transmitted from Animals to Man*: 147-173. Springfield IL: C. C. Thomas.

Drancourt, M. and D. Raoult. 2002. Molecular insights into the history of plague. *Microbes and Infection* 4(1): 105-109.

Dzierzykray-Rogalski, T. and E. Prominska. 1994. A further report on Pharaoh Siptah's handicap (XIXth Egyptian Dynasty). *HOMO* 45 (Supplement), S45.

Ebbell, B. 1937. *The Papyrus Ebers.* Copenhagen: Levin and Munksgaard.

Geller, M. J. 2010. *Ancient Babylonian Medicine: Theory and Practice.* Oxford: Wiley-Blackwell.

Goedicke, H. 1984. The Canaanite Illness. *Studien zur Altägyptischen Kultur* 11: 91-105.

Györy, H. 2010. *J3dt rnpt* or the 'Pestilence of the Year', in J. Cockitt and R. David (eds.) *Pharmacy and Medicine in Ancient Egypt: Proceedings of the Conferences Held in Cairo (2007) and Manchester (2008)*: 81-84. Oxford: Archaeopress.

Hoffmeier, J. K. 1996. *Israel in Egypt: The Evidence for the Authenticity of the Exodus Tradition.* Oxford: Oxford University Press.

Hopkins, D. 1980. Ramses V: earliest known victim? *World Health* (May): 220.

Hoyte, H. M. 1993. The plagues of Egypt: what killed the animals and the firstborn? *Medical Journal of Australia* 158(10): 285-286.

Kozloff, A. P. 2006. Bubonic plague during the reign of Amenhotep III. *KMT* 17(3): 36-46.

Leitz, C. 2000. *Magical and Medical Papyri of the New Kingdom.* London: British Museum Press.

Marr, J. S. and C. D. Malloy, 1996. An epidemiologic analysis of the ten plagues of Egypt. *Caduceus* 12(1): 7-24.

Miller, R. L., S. Ikram, G. J. Armelagos, R. Walker, W. B. Harer and C. J. Schiff. 1994. Diagnosis of *Plasmodium falciparum* infection in mummies using the Rapid Manual *Para*Sight™-F test. *Transactions of the Royal Society of Tropical Medicine and Hygiene* 88: 31-32.

Mitchell, J. K. 1900. Study of a mummy affected with anterior poliomyelitis. *Philadelphia Medical Journal* 6: 414-415.

Møller-Christensen, V. and D. R. Hughes. 1966. An early case of leprosy in Nubia. *Man* 1:242-243.

Moran, W. L. 1992. *The Amarna Letters.* Baltimore: John Hopkins University Press.

Nunn, J. F. 1996. *Ancient Egyptian Medicine*: 95. London: British Museum Press.

Panagiotakopulu, E. 2004. Pharaonic Egypt and the origins of plague. *Journal of Biogeography* 31: 269-275.

Ruffer, M. A. and A. R. Ferguson 1911. Note on an eruption resembling that of variola in the skin of a mummy of the XXth Dynasty. *Journal of Pathology and Bacteriology* 15: 1-3.

Rutherford, P. 2008. DNA identification in mummies and associated material, in R. David (ed.) *Egyptian Mummies and Modern Science:* 116-132. Cambridge: Cambridge University Press.

Sallares, G., S. Gomzi, A. Richards, and C. Anderung. 2000. Evidence from ancient DNA for malaria in antiquity. Abstract in *Proceedings of the 5th International Ancient DNA Conference, Manchester.*

Sandison, A. T. 1972. Evidence of infectious diseases. *Journal of Human Evolution* 1: 213-214.

Smith, G. E. 1912. *The Royal Mummies.* Catalogue général des antiquités égyptiennes du Musée du Caire. Cairo: Imprimerie de l'Institut français d'archéologie orientale.

Strouhal, E. 1996. Traces of smallpox epidemic in the family of Ramses V of the Egyptian 20th Dynasty. *Anthropologie* 34: 315-319.

Tiradritti, F. 2014. Of kilns and corpses: Theban plague victims. *Egyptian Archaeology* 44: 15-18.

Application of Oils and Resins During the Process of Mummification: Experimental Analysis and Study Problems

Laura García-Jiménez

laugarciajimenez@gmail.com
Department of Egyptology, Complutense University of Madrid

Abstract: The embalmers that carried out the mummification applied several substances during the different steps in order to preserve the body and to secure eternity in the afterlife.

These materials applied during the process of mummification have presented problems when identifying their typology and how they were employed. The cedar oil and the resin provide two examples. Since the 19th century researchers have studied the Egyptian papyri and the Classical authors, but there are still unknown words or misinterpretations. The science advances, and from the middle of the 20th century onwards, studies about the possible materials were more exhaustive, analyzing the mummies themselves as source of knowledge. Experiments have always been a good way to see the reality of theories with our own eyes.

Thus, with the experiment that I conducted in 2014, applying the three methods describe by Herodotus to three rabbits, I saw the reality of the problem regarding which substances to apply. Therefore I compared the classical authors as Herodotus, Diodorus and Pliny among others, and I gathered information from the research of the two last centuries, highlighting Lucas, Garner, Ikram and Brier as empirical investigation; and Abdel-Maksoud, Buckley, Nerlich, Zink and others as laboratory research.

The fact that some substances are volatile or of unknown origin is one of the many limitations for their study, but thanks to new technologies, we can begin to clarify some of the doubts that had arisen.

The objective is to expose all these doubts and hypotheses, compare them with the results and conclusions of my experiment, and finally to present a modern image of the possible embalming products.

Keywords: mummification, materials, oil, resin, experiment

Introduction

Mummification for the ancient Egyptians was one of the fundamental steps by which to reach the eternal life. They were constantly improving this technical process and gaining new methods, for which they needed a knowledge of the human body and also of what substances to apply and the techniques involved. Both questions in some cases continue to be a riddle for us. We must keep in mind that neither medicine nor the use of substances in humans were static for millennia, either to cure a disease or, in our case, to carry out a mummification.

Sources

Ancient Egyptian Sources

A known Egyptian description of the technical processes involved in mummification does not exist. Papyri are preserved which fragmentary information and artistic representations, but

Pharmacy and Medicine in Ancient Egypt
(Archaeopress 2021): 15–29

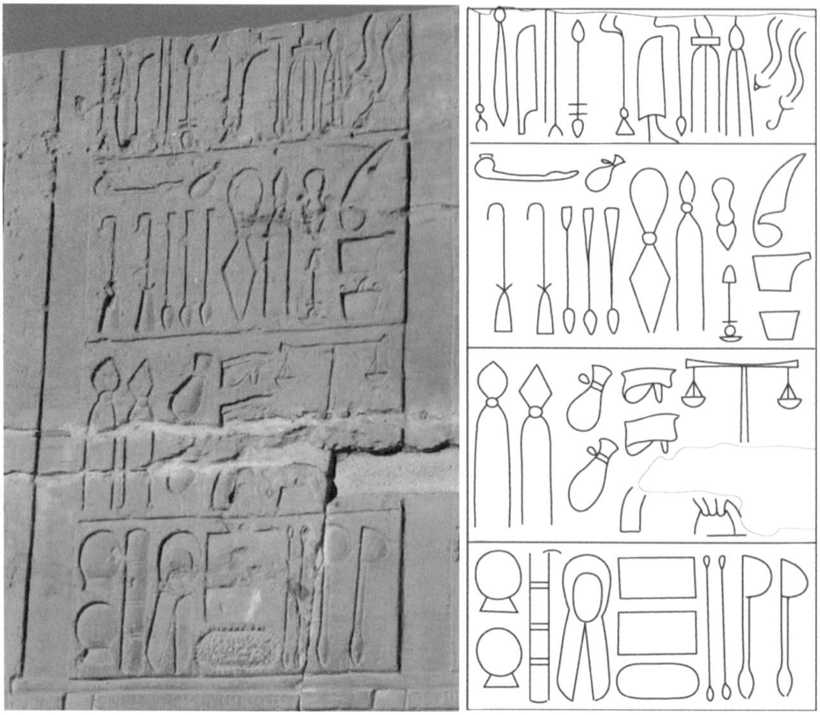

Fig. 1. Photograph and drawing of the Kom Ombo surgical instrument scene
(Coppens 2010, pp. 128-129)

taken as a whole these pictorial and written description contain no real details with regard to the actual mechanics of mummification.

Papyri

We have fragments of medical papyri such as the Ebers papyrus whose content can help us better understand mummification also in relation to the materials and processes that were used.

Ebers papyrus is preserved today in Leipzig and is the longest of the extant medical papyri at approximately 20 meters. It consists of 110 pages and 887 paragraphs, many of them with magical content. It was purchased in 1862 in Luxor, and dates from the 18th dynasty, but it is likely that it was a copy of a text from the Old Kingdom, it has been suggested that it came from the tomb of a doctor. It was translated into English for the first time from the hieratic by Ghalioungui (1987). We may also highlight a monograph about this papyrus and its content by Bryan in 1930 (Nunn 2002, pp. 30-34).

This and other medical papyri provide us with a lot of Egyptian words for plants and substances used as medicinal remedies. The ancient Egyptians being aware of the pharmacological properties that could be applied in the steps of mummification, and in these cases, among the most clearly identified botanical species are:

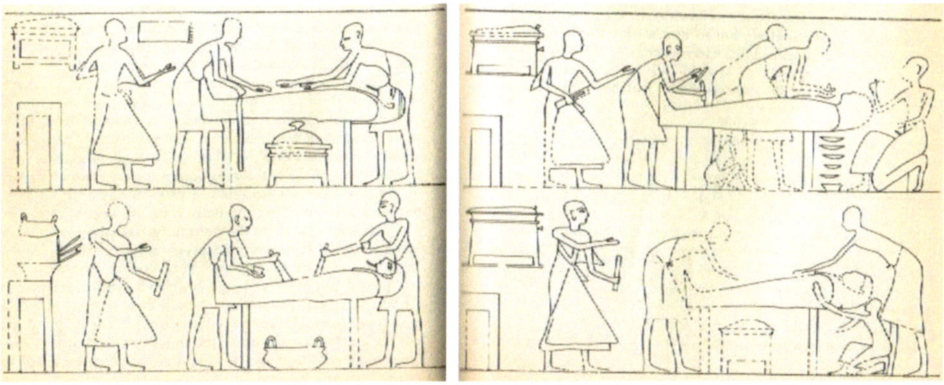

Fig. 2. Tomb of Thay (Spencer 1982, pp. 132-133)

- *Juniperus phoenicea* as an antiseptic would reduce the possibility of infection or putrefaction, also used only in live patients as diuretic, carminative (facilitating eructation), styptic (astringent that causes contraction of tissues and prevention of bleeding and secretion), and anodyne relieving pain (Nunn 2002, p. 215).
- *Ricinus communis* can be used as a powerful purgative, and can also be externally applied as a demulcent, soothing and relieving irritation (Nunn 2002, p. 216).

Including not only medicines of plant origin, but also mineral or animal:

- Natron (*hesmen*), a compound of sodium chloride, sulphate, carbonate, and bicarbonate induces vomiting and absorbs moisture (Nunn 2002, p. 145) and is used in mummification as desiccant of the body[1].
- Honey (*bit*), used as an antibacterial substance with fungal properties (Nunn 2002, p. 148; Zimmerman 2017, p. 148)

Artistic representations

Along with the knowledge provided by the papyri, we find pictures in tombs, temples or coffins that can provide us with a more accurate idea. Outstanding examples:

- On the walls of the Temples of Edfu and Dendera, of the Ptolemaic Period, is a list of the ingredients that were used during the ritual where the offerings were prepared (Pujol 2004); and at the Temple of Kom Ombo can be found the first representation of medical instruments for performing surgery, possibly extrapolated to their use in dead bodies (Coppens 2010, pp. 128-129) (Fig. 1).
- The 19th Dynasty Theban Tombs TT 23 of Thay (Fig. 2) and TT 41 of Amenemopet (Fig. 3) show the anointing and wrapping of the body as well as the preparation of grave goods (Spencer 1982, pp. 132-134).

1 From Wadi Natrum in Egypt, for its state and timing of application in mummification and more information about natron: Lucas, A 1914, 'The Use of Natron by the Ancient Egyptian in Mummification', *JEA* 1, pp. 119–123; and Lucas, A and Harris, JR 1999, *Ancient Egyptian Materials and Industries*, Mineola, New York, Dover Publications, pp. 297-303.

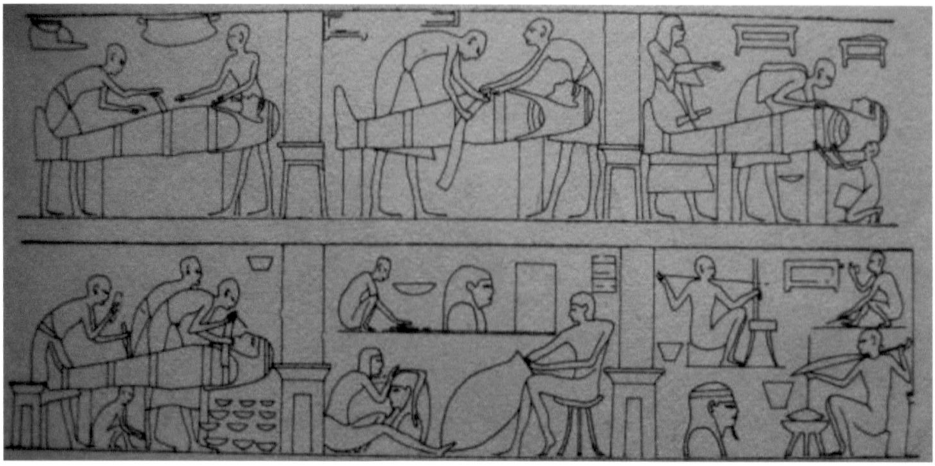

Fig. 3. Tomb of Amenemopet (Spencer 1982, p. 134)

- The anthropomorphic coffin of Dyedbastiufanj (Djed-bastet-iuef-ankh), from the Ptolemaic era, displayed in the Museum of Hildesheim, contains bandage and ritualistic scenes (Soria, n.d.)

Instruments found in caches have expanded our knowledge and we know of different elongated iron or copper objects, whose end can have a hook, both curved and curly, or a kind of spoon; spacers to keep the incision open; tweezers; enemas; bowls of all kinds (some of wood to withstand the heat of the resins); likewise jars and containers of all sizes, etc. Even embalming stone tables have been found with holes and corresponding inclination so that the blood does not stagnate (Janot 1996)

Greek and Roman authors

With Egyptian sources containing scant information regarding mummification, Greek and Roman authors become the main source. We have to be careful not to take these writings literally because they are based on oral transmission or through previous Classical authors.

Herodotus in *Histories* (Book II) (Godley 1920, pp. 370-373) described three methods of mummification according to social status, making reference to certain materials that we want to highlight: 1) Palm wine and aromatics (myrrh, cinnamon and others except frankincense) that would serve to wash the intestines; natrum, in which the body is covered for 70 days to dry; linen for bandaging; and gum to anoint as if it were glue. 2) Cedar oil, applied with an enema to fill the abdomen, liquefying the viscera; and natrum as above. 3) To clean out the intestines a clyster (possibly water) was used; and again natrum as above.

II, 86. '[...] The mode of embalming, according to the most perfect process, is the following: They take first a crooked piece of iron, and with it draw out the brain through the nostrils, thus getting rid of a portion, while the skull is cleared of the rest by rinsing with drugs; next they make a cut along the flank with a sharp Ethiopian stone, and take out the whole contents of the abdomen, which they then cleanse, washing it thoroughly with palm wine, and again frequently with an infusion of pounded aromatics. After this they fill the cavity with the purest bruised myrrh, with cassia, and every other sort of spicery except frankincense, and sew up the opening. Then the body is placed in natrum for seventy days, and covered entirely over. After the expiration of that space of time, which must not be exceeded, the body is washed, and wrapped round, from head to foot, with bandages of fine linen cloth, smeared over with gum, which is used generally by the Egyptians in the place of glue, and in this state it is given back to the relations, who enclose it in a wooden case which they have had made for the purpose, shaped into the figure of a man. Then fastening the case, they place it in a sepulchral chamber, upright against the wall. Such is the most costly way of embalming the dead'.

II, 87. 'If persons wish to avoid expense, and choose the second process, the following is the method pursued: Syringes are filled with oil made from the cedar-tree, which is then, II, 86. '[...] The mode of embalming, according to the most perfect process, is the following: They take first a crooked piece of iron, and with it draw out the brain through the nostrils, thus getting rid of a portion, while the skull is cleared of the rest by rinsing with drugs; next they make a cut along the flank with a sharp Ethiopian stone, and take out the whole contents of the abdomen, which they then cleanse, washing it thoroughly with palm wine, and again frequently with an infusion of pounded aromatics. After this they fill the cavity with the purest bruised myrrh, with cassia, and every other sort of spicery except frankincense, and sew up the opening. Then the body is placed in natrum for seventy days, and covered entirely over. After the expiration of that space of time, which must not be exceeded, the body is washed, and wrapped round, from head to foot, with bandages of fine linen cloth, smeared over with gum, which is used generally by the Egyptians in the place of glue, and in this state it is given back to the relations, who enclose it in a wooden case which they have had made for the purpose, shaped into the figure of a man. Then fastening the case, they place it in a sepulchral chamber, upright against the wall. Such is the most costly way of embalming the dead'.

II, 87. 'If persons wish to avoid expense, and choose the second process, the following is the method pursued: Syringes are filled with oil made from the cedar-tree, which is then, without any incision or disembowelling, injected into the abdomen. The passage by which it might be likely to return is stopped, and the body laid in natrum the prescribed number of days. At the end of the time the cedar-oil is allowed to make its escape; and such is its power that it brings with it the whole stomach and intestines in a liquid state. The natrum meanwhile has dissolved the flesh, and so nothing is left of the dead body but the skin and the bones. It is returned in this condition to the relatives, without any further trouble being bestowed upon it'.

II, 88. 'The third method of embalming, which is practised in the case of the poorer classes, is to clear out the intestines with a clyster, and let the body lie in natrum the seventy days, after which it is at once given to those who come to fetch it away'.

Diodorus Siculus in *Library of History* (vol. 1) (Oldfather 1933, pp. 309-313) also named three methods but only explained the first, commenting on the family tradition of the embalmer's profession and the costs. The substances quoted are: Palm wine and spices to wash the intestines; Cedar oil together with myrrh and cinnamon anointed for 30 days to preserve and give a good smell.

> I, 91, 5 [...] 'When they have gathered to treat the body after it has been slit open, one of them thrusts his hand through the opening in the corpse into the trunk and extracts everything but the kidneys and heart, and another one cleanses each of the viscera, washing them in palm wine and spices. [6] And in general, they carefully dress the whole body for over thirty days, first with cedar oil and certain other preparations, and then with myrrh, cinnamon, and such spices as have the faculty not only of preserving it for a long time but also of giving it a fragrant odour. And after treating the body they return it to the relatives of the deceased, every member of it having been so preserved intact that even the hair on the eyelids and brows remains, the entire appearance of the body is unchanged, and the cast of its shape is recognizable' [...]

Strabo in Book 16 of his Geography alluded to the asphalt used to embalm bodies, like a type of resin (Hamilton 1903, pp. 184).

> XVI, 45. 'The Egyptians use the *asphaltus* for embalming the bodies of the dead'

Pliny wrote that Syrian Cedar was the *cedrium* with which people were embalmed in Egypt. (Rackham 1945, p. 420)

> XVI, 52. 'In Europe tar is obtained from the torch-pine by heating it, and is used for coating ships' tackle and many other purposes. The wood of the tree is chopped up and put into ovens and heated by means of a fire packed all round outside. The first liquid that exudes flows like water down a pipe; in Syria this is called *cedrium*, and it is so strong that in Egypt it is used for embalming the bodies of the dead'

Modern studies

Researchers from the **beginning of the 20th century** began to publish more specific studies of substances, materials, and instruments, as well as their applications in the process of mummification, forming a consensus about their chronological and technical evolution.

Chemist Alfred Lucas was ones of the most important researchers of materials, publishing in the first third of the century articles on bitumen (1914) and cedar (1931) among others, and in 1933 published a monograph on materials and substances, laying the foundations for later books like Lucas and Harris (1999) and Nicholson and Shaw (2000).

The century progressed and **multidisciplinary projects** with studies of mummies appeared. In Manchester, the work of Rosalie David and her team (1972-1984) and also the Canadian project led by the Cockburns (1980) were studies about materials and substances that had relevance in the mummification process.

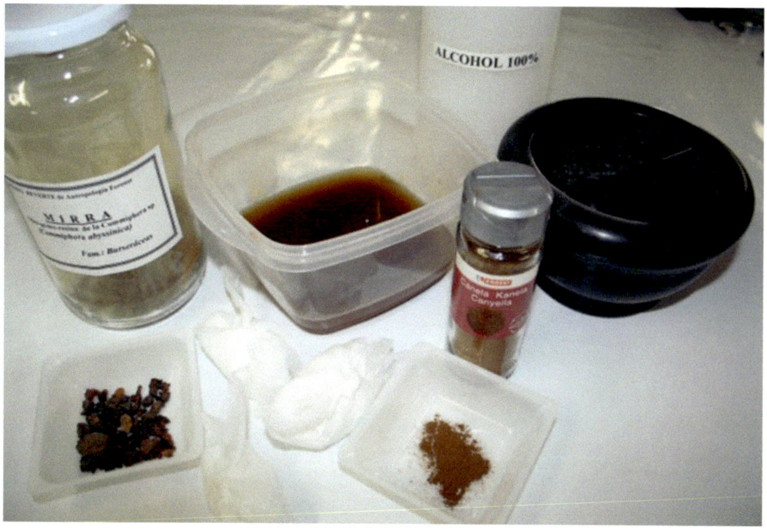

Fig. 4. 'Palm wine' made by us using it in the Method I (Photography by Laura García 2014)

As one of the pioneer studies in this field we may highlight the work of Iskander and Zaki in 1943, and as the first work that used modern chemical techniques on previously studied materials, the work of Buckley and Evershed (2001) stands out.

Modern scientific **analysis of mummies** now proliferates, and we can extract more information. But it is true that some processes or uses of materials remain beyond our understanding and we are not sure what was used or how. It is for this reason that empirical studies are so important, applying all the knowledge we have and trying to extract information to refute or verify some of the issues for which we still have no answer.

The first **experimental mummification** was carried out by Robert **Garner** in 1979, as part of the Manchester Museum Mummy Project directed by Rosalie David, applying to rats some mummification methods with materials such as cedar oil.

Brier and Wade (2001), in 1994, went further with the 'Mumab Project', since they wanted to apply the most complete mummification process that was known and to simulate the ancients Egyptians. They made replicas of instruments, containers, embalming table and *ushebtis*, and acquired spices and oils from present-day Egypt, completing the first human mummification in 2000 years.

Ikram (2005) in the 'Animal Mummy Project' performed different mummification methods and applied different materials to be able to compare the results in several animals. The resin, wax, incense, oils and linen were easily purchased, but palm wine was more problematic and a local gin had to be used. And although there was an initial attempt to reproduce cedar, pine or juniper oil, in the event lettuce and castor oil were used, which were produced in antiquity as they are today.

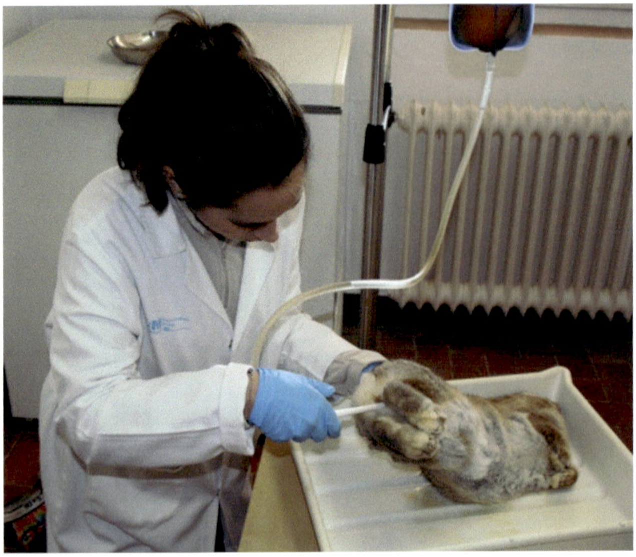

Fig. 5. Applying 'cedar oil' *per anum* with a drip enema (Photography by Mercedes González 2014)

Finally, we may add my **own empirical study**_made in 2014 with the help of Mercedes Gonzalez, director of Instituto de Estudios Científicos en Momias (IECIM) in Madrid. It was conducted following the three methods described by Herodotus, applying them on three different rabbits. In the matter of materials and instruments, some originals were collected such as the stone of Ethiopia, natron, linen, Arabic gum or myrrh. Within the possibilities, we tried to reproduce even the most doubtful substances faithfully using, for example, for the 'palm wine' a liquor, ethanol and spices (cinnamon and myrrh), and for the 'cedar oil' enema, oil of cedar with guaiacol and sunflower oil.

All of these studies and experiments presented a lot of new conclusions, disputing theories and raising new questions about mummification, its procedures and the materials themselves.

Doubts and problems about substances and materials during the process of mummification

The main problem is the lack of data. There is no Egyptian papyrus that explains in detail the techniques used to embalm, either because it has not been preserved or found or maybe because knowledge was transmitted orally from teacher-father to apprentice-child as Diodorus suggests (I, 91, 6). There are a few references that basically deal with the religious aspect. We have the Ritual of Embalming, translated by Sauneron (1952), its most complete version is preserved on Papyrus Boulaq 3, dated to the mid first century AD. It can be considered a methodological manual that emphasizes religious or magical formulas and from which we have only the description of the last part of mummification since the beginning stages are missing.

More technical information has provided the Apis Embalming Ritual preserved on Papyrus Vindob 3873, dating to the second half of second century BC. This details almost the entire ritual period of mummification (Chapman 2017).

The different interpretations of the sparse information available about the process is other inconvenience. In Classical writings one of the problems is decontextualization, because they can be misinterpreted by not taking into account the origin of testimonies and which were factual and which were not. The translations made throughout the century, have been able to distort or change original statements. And also, substances were ignored and were not valued as sources of information until the appearance of modern methods that made their study possible.

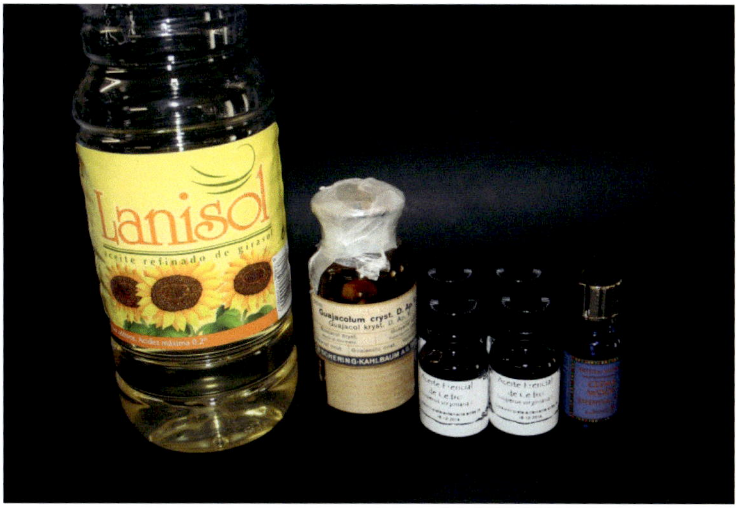

Fig. 6. 'Cedar oil' made by us using it in the Method II (Photography by Laura García 2014)

But we are able to make different interpretations in the papyri too, since we are uncertain of the meaning of many Egyptian words. For example, of about 160 medicines obtained from plants only about 20% have been identified with certainty, either because we don't know their translation or what they were referring specifically to (Zimmerman 2017, p. 148).

The material itself creates confusion in various aspects:

- In its typology or origin, when scientists try to identify the type of plant, they sometimes compare it with current ones, but flora and fauna of thousands of years ago have changed. And the same applies to investigations about where it came from, if it was native or if it was imported, relating it to domestic and foreign trade.
- In its function or application, since different functions may have different application methods, and with certain substances there is uncertainty about techniques for use or what it would be used for.
- In its dating, since it is difficult to know when a material began to be used due to variation over time, the use of different materials for a certain function, or even if it was only used in a specific place and time.
- And in its evidence, since depending on source, the technical process and materials used can be confusing or contradictory for us.

Materials used during the process of mummification

Resin may be extracted from coniferous trees such as cedar, juniper or pine. But given coniferous trees are not native to Egypt, it would be an imported material from Hit-Abu (Iraq) or from south of Egypt. 'Arabic gum', another type of resin was also used and was obtained from the *pistacia* tree in some cases. And in mineral form, 'tar' and 'pitch' can be used interchangeably, both are applied to viscous materials of asphalt or bitumen (Bahn 1992, p. 109; Lucas and Harris 1999, p. 317).

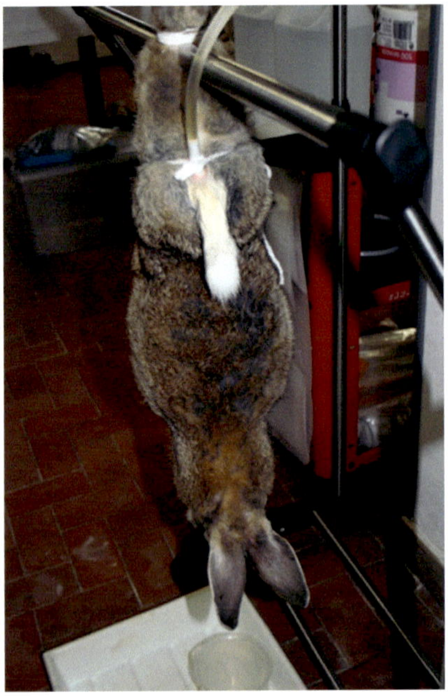

Fig. 7. Drip enema of water in the Method III (Photography by Laura García 2014)

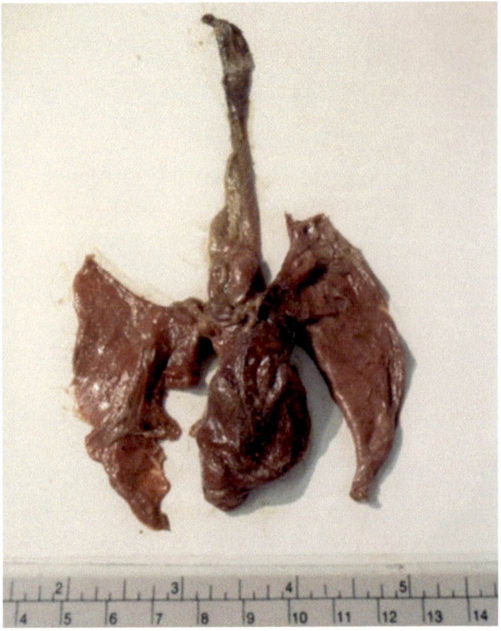

Fig. 8. Trachea, lungs and heart of rabbit Method II perfectly preserved. After 70 days with the cedar oil enema inside and the body in natron (Photography by Laura García 2014)

The function was not only to conserve but also to carry out an antimicrobial action. So molten 'resin' (although conifers are very resistant to fire) would serve as a filling of the cranial cavity to give flexibility after drying and moving the limbs; and it could also be used in solid added form within the permanent filling's sacks (Abdel-Maksoud and El-Armin 2011, pp. 132-142; Dawson 1927, p. 46). Molten 'Arabic gum' could serve as an adhesive for bandage. And we know that the 'tar' anointed on the body displaced in the last moments of mummification the natrum as a desiccant element (Aufderheide *et al.* 2004, p. 65).

Regarding dating, we have remains of resin on bandages since Neolithic period. For example, pine resin was found in a mummy located in Mostagedda and analysed by Jones and Buckley (2014). And in the Ptolemaic period tar was used prominently as a preservative and desiccant, hence the black skin appearance of mummies that have come down to us.

We have evidence that resin was used during the process of mummification. It was discovered both in the classical sources as well as in the residues inside jars and even within the mummies themselves. In fact it is curious that the Persian word for bitumen is *mummia*. (Bahn 1992, p. 109).

Cedar oil is another main substance and as its name indicates that it could have come from the cedar tree. Nevertheless there are doubts regarding which tree would be used to extract this 'Cedar oil' cited in the classical writings. Egypt didn't have a high variety of trees, and imported a great deal of cedar from Phoenicia (modern Lebanon). However, it is possible that

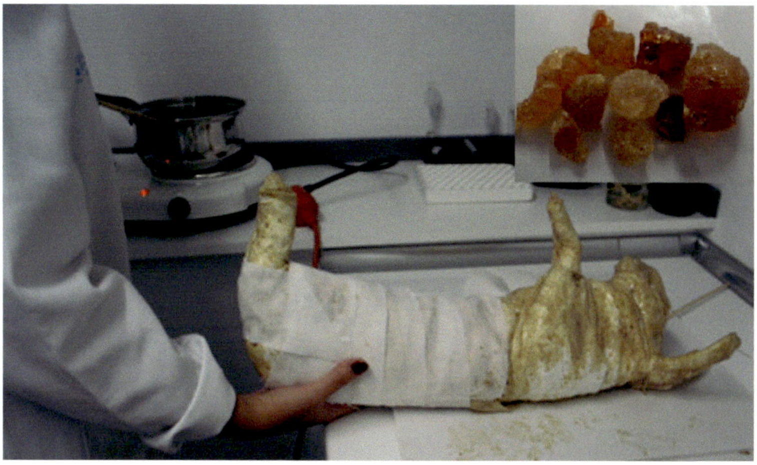

Fig. 9. Arabic gum applied in Method II (and in I and II too) after melting in ceramic hob (Photography by Mercedes González 2014).

another coniferous tree such as juniper or pine was used or even that it was actually turpentine obtained from the distillation of conifer resin, mostly pine (Lucas 1931).

Applying cedar oil as enema *per anum*, the purpose would be to liquefy the organs and thus facilitate their extraction. This could happen using turpentine which even today is mainly used as a dissolvent. And would serve to conserve because its main component is guaiacol. To apply it on the skin, would act not only as a preservative also as a perfumed oil that would leave a good smell. (Ikram 2005, pp. 37-38).

We have Herodotus and Diodorus' testimonies that named the cedar oil, relating it to theories of Mediterranean *Juniperus oxicedrus*, which is really a juniper. And it is true that even the cedar oil that we use today comes from another juniper, the *Juniperus Virginiana* of America. Pliny also mentioned the *cedrium*, which could be related to the pine turpentine to liquefy, as with Herodotus, while the cedar oil mentioned by Diodorus would have more relation to use in anointing (Koller *et al.* 2005, p. 619; Lucas 1930, p. 45).

Palm wine is an alcoholic product from the sap of a palm tree, nevertheless, despite its literal denomination, it has also been related to the vine. Liquid would be applied to clean the abdomen after removing the viscera and/or to wash them. It was a volatile substance and hardly detectable in mummies, although Herodotus and Diodorus commented on its function and the moment of application in the process of mummification (Lucas and Harris 1999, p. 316). We also have artistic representations with vine and palm scenes, but not linked to embalming scenes[2].

Beeswax is an animal product, whose function was to preserve and to be an antibacterial and hydrophobic agent. It had many applications, such as to cover bodily orifices as ears, eyes, mouth or ventral incision; smear the body as a resin ('black wax'); or seal linen bandages as

2 More information about scenes of viticulture and winemaking in Ancient Egypt analysed in research Project 'Irep en Kemet' directed by Dr. Guasch: www.wineofancientegypt.com

an adhesive (Lucas and Harris 1999, p. 303). Thus honey and beeswax have been represented throughout the history of ancient Egypt. There are hieroglyphs with bees as *bîty* that form part of the royal title *nsw-bîty*, meaning the 'King of the dualities' or King of Upper and Lower Egypt (Collier and Manley 2000, p. 43). And also there are artistic representations with scenes of honey extraction in beehives in tombs; in these cases the owner's titles were related to these functions, for example Tomb of Pasaba, a honey collector. Moreover, as a curiosity, the Coptic word 'mum' means wax (Buckley and Evershed 2001, p. 840).

Aromatic substances were numerous, although we have evidence of few of them. Since the classical period, cinnamon or myrrh were related to the process of mummification, and it is possible that the cassia of the ancient Egyptians, mentioned by Herodotus, should be related to modern cinnamon which Diodorus cited. Myrrh, added to a gum that gave smell, could also be used as an ointment, while other times, this and other aromatics could be used as incense (Lucas 1930, pp. 47-50).

Application of the materials and substances in the experiment

Once we had investigated the sources, limitations and materials used during the process of mummification, the next step in this research was to analyse the reaction of some of these substances and materials in our own empirical study. As previously mentioned, to each rabbit was applied one of the three methods described by Herodotus, and in each of them, different substances were used.

In Method I, the most expensive according to Herodotus, were used materials such as Ethiopian stone to make the ventral incision, natron for desiccation, palm wine to wash the cavity and the viscera extracted, cinnamon and myrrh as aromatics, linen for bandaging and Arabic gum used as adhesive. Regarding 'Palm wine', we made it with 50ml of liquor mixed with 30% of alcohol, 500ml of ethanol and aromatics (cinnamon and myrrh); we used it as a disinfectant. (Fig. 4)

In Method II, cedar oil was applied *per anum* with a drip enema (Fig. 5) to liquefy internal organs and then check if it was possible to extract them. This 'Cedar oil' was composed of 47ml of cedar essential oil, 45ml of guaiacol and 530ml of sunflower oil, in total 622ml (Fig. 6). In relation to desiccation, salt and sodium bicarbonate were used for drying, instead of natron.

And in Method III, we also used a drip enema *per anum* but 500ml of distilled water were introduced with the intention of purging (Fig. 7).

Results

During the experiment, in relation to the substances, we encountered a few problems. In the case of the 'palm wine', as a volatile substance and almost undetectable in mummies, it is difficult to know the origin, palm tree or vine, so we finally decided to use marc, a liquor that would provide a sufficient percentage of alcohol to serve as a disinfectant, achieving the same goal as the Egyptians when washing the organs.

We realized that essential cedar oil is denser than previously we thought, so we had to heat it with own hands, having even to heat one of the tins with water at 40° for an easier introduction. This introduction had to be gradual, so we had to position the rabbit upside down. It is difficult to understand how Egyptians could achieve this. Regarding the 622ml of 'cedar oil', we were only able to introduce 582ml into the body, enlarging the diameter of the rabbit from 38cm to 45cm. And the end, it didn't fulfill our purpose, since it didn't liquefy the viscera although it could be that it conserved them (Fig. 8).

Regarding the water used in the third method, there were two possible objectives: to liquefy or to purge, and neither was fulfilled. This was because it didn't liquefy the organs before decomposition arrived, and because it is not possible to use an enema after death, since the peristaltic movements of the intestine cease, but we don't know if in Ancient Egypt this was achieved with pressure.

Also, another result to highlight is Arabic gum, since melted it worked as an adhesive to fix the linen bandages, but the problem appeared when we wanted to melt it and finally we had to turn to a ceramic hob, leaving us with the mystery of how the Egyptians would do it (Fig. 9).

Conclusions

After many setbacks during the experiment and after analyzing past studies, one of the main conclusions was to consider our ignorance about some aspects of ancient Egyptian knowledge in relation to mummification. We must be careful when we assume what materials were used and how were employed. In this case, we decided to use Arabic gum as a possible resin, due to its antiquity and easy dissolution. Nevertheless we discovered that this dissolution was not so simple, even so, it is valid as an adhesive when it is melted.

There is also controversy regarding 'cedar oil', since we didn't know if it was really cedar, juniper, pine or other type of conifer. We can, however, confirm that it worked as a good preservative, since cedar oil stopped or slowed down decomposition during drying, and surely organs dried before they rotted.

Finally, regarding processes, in Methods II and III it's clear that enemas didn't achieve their objectives. In Method II, organs didn't liquefy and exit the body *per anum*, and in Method III a purge was not possible. Classical texts may have been misunderstood, or simply, we don't know the process used.

We know that there are many questions unanswered but the objective is to show the many different aspects that are pending and that remain to be researched. And this is and will be possible thanks to the collaboration between humanities and sciences, being able to take new perspectives, helping in the experiment to visualize these ancient practices and give truth to theories.

Bibliography

Classical authors:

Diodorus Siculus 1933, *Library of History, Volume I: Books 1-2.34.* Translated by C. H. Oldfather, Loeb Classical Library 279, Harvard University Press, Cambridge, MA.

Herodotus 1920, *The Persian Wars, Volume I: Books 1-2*, translated by A. D. Godley, Loeb Classical Library 117, Harvard University Press, Cambridge, MA.

Pliny 1945, *Natural History, Volume IV: Books 12-16*, Translated by H. Rackham, Loeb Classical Library 370, Harvard University Press, Cambridge, MA.

Strabo 1903, *Geography*, translated by H. C. Hamilton, George Bell & Sons, London.

Modern:

Abdel-Maksoud, G and El-Armin, AR 2011, 'A Review on the Materials used during the Mummification Processes in Ancient Egypt', *Mediterranean Archaeology and Archaeometry*, vol. 1, no. 2, pp. 129–150.

Aufderheide, AC, Cartmell, L, Zlonis, M and Sheldrick, P 2004, 'Mummification practices at Kellis site in Egypt's Dakhleh Oasis', *Journal of the Society for the Study of Egyptian Antiquities (JSSEA)*, vol. 31, pp. 63–77.

Bahn, P 1992, 'The Making a Mummy', *Nature*, vol. 356, p. 109.

Brier, B and Wade, R 2001, 'Surgical Procedures during Ancient Egyptian Mummification', *Chungara*, vol. 33, pp. 117–123.

Bryan, CP 1930, *Ancient Egyptian Medicine. The Papyrus Ebers*, Ares Publishers, London.

Buckley, S and Evershed, R 2001, 'Organic Chemistry of embalming agent in Pharaonic and Graeco-Roman mummies', *Nature*, vol. 413, pp. 837–841.

Chapman, SL 2017, 'The Embalming Ritual of the Late Period through Ptolemaic Egypt', PhD. University of Birmingham.

Cockburn, A and Cockburn, E (eds) 1980, *Mummies, disease and Ancient Cultures*, Cambridge University Press, Cambridge.

Collier, M and Manley, B (eds) 2000, *Introducción a los Jeroglíficos egipcios*. Translated by J.R. Pérez-Accino, Alianza Editorial, Madrid.

David, AR (ed) 1979, *The Manchester Museum Mummy Project*, Manchester University Press, Manchester.

Dawson, WR 1927, 'Making a Mummy', *Journal of Egyptian Archaeology (JEA)*, vol. 13, pp. 40–49.

Engelbach, R and Derry, D 1942, 'Mummufication', *Annales du Service des antiquités de l'Egypte (ASAE)*, vol. 41, pp. 233–265.

Garner, R 1979, 'Experimental mummification', in David, AR (ed), *The Manchester Museum Mummy Project*, Manchester Museum, Manchester, pp. 19-24.

Ghalioungui, P 1969, 'Early specialization in Ancient Egyptian Medicine and its possible relation to an archetypal image of the human organism', *Medical History*, vol. 13, no. 4, pp. 382-386.

Ghalioungui, P 1987, *The Ebers Papyrus: A New English Translation, Commentaries and Glossaries*, Academy of Scientific Research and Technology, Cairo.

Ikram, S 2005, 'Manufacturing Divinity: The Technology of Mummification', in Ikram, I (ed), *Divine Creatures. Animal Mummies in Ancient Egypt*, The American University in Cairo Press, Cairo, New York, pp. 16–43

Iskander, Z and Shaheen, A 1964, 'Temporary Stuffing Materials used in the Process of Mummification in Ancient Egypt', *Annales du Service des antiquités de l'Egypte (ASAE)*, vol. 58, pp. 197–208.

Iskander, Z and Zaki, A 1943, 'Materials and Method used for mummifying the body of Amentenekht, Saqqara 1941', *Annales du Service des antiquités de l'Egypte (ASAE)*, vol. 42, pp. 223–250.

Janot, F 1996, 'Les instruments et la pratique des prêtres-embaumeurs, *Le Bulletin de l'Institut français d'archéologie orientale (BIFAO)*, vol. 96, pp. 245-253.

Jones, J, Higham, T, Oldfield, R, O'Connor, T and Buckley, SA 2014, 'Evidence for Prehistoric Origins of Egyptian Mummification in Late Neolithic Burials', *PLOS ONE*, vol. 9, pp. 1–13.

Koller, J, Baumer, U, Kaup, Y and Weser, U 2005, 'Herodotus' and Pliny's embalming materials identified on ancient Egyptian Mummies', *Archaeometry*, vol. 47, pp. 609–628.

Koller, J, Baumer, U, Kaup, Y, Schmid, M and Weser, U, 2003, 'Effective Mummification Compounds Used in Pharaonic Egypt: Reactivity on Bone Alkaline Phosphatase', *Z. Naturforsch,* vol. 58b, pp. 462-480.

Lucas, A 1930, 'Cosmetics, Perfumes and Inciense in ancient Egypt', *Journal of Egyptian Archaeology (JEA),* vol. 16, pp. 41–53.

Lucas, A 1931, "Cedar'-tree products employed in mummification', *Journal of Egyptian Archaeology (JEA),* vol. 17, pp. 13–21.

Lucas, A and Harris, JR 1999, *Ancient Egyptian Materials and Industries*, Dover Publications Mineola, New York.

Millet, NB, Hart, GD, Reyman, TA, Zimmerman, MR and Lewin PK 1980, 'ROM I: mummification for the common people', in Cockburn, A and Cockburn, E (eds), *Mummies, Disease and Ancient Cultures*, Cambridge University Press, Cambridge, pp. 71–84.

Nicholson, PT and Shaw, I (eds) 2000, *Ancient Egyptian Materials and Technology*, Cambridge University Press, Cambridge.

Nunn, JF 2002, *Ancient Egyptian Medicine*, University of Oklahoma Press, Oklahoma.

Pujol, R 2004, 'El Perfume en el Antiguo Egipto. Amigos de la Egiptología', viewed 05 September 2019, <http://www.egiptologia.com/content/view/513/45/1/2/>

Reyman, TA and Peck, WH 1980, 'Egyptian mummification with evisceration per ano', in Cockburn, A &Cockburn, E (eds), *Mummies, Disease and Ancient Cultures.* Cambridge, pp. 85-100.

Sauneron, S 1952, *Rituel de l'embaumement: Pap. Boulaq III, Pap. Louvre 5.158*, Imprimerie Nationale: Service des Antiquités de l'Égypte, Caire.

Soria, T (n.d.), 'La Momificación en el Antiguo Egipto: Origen, Fuentes, Técnicas y Estudios Modernos de las Momias Egipcias', viewed 05 September 2019, <http://www.egiptomania.com/mitologia/momificacion.htm>

Spencer, AJ 1982, *Death in Ancient Egypt*, Penguin Books, London.

Zimmerman, M 2017, 'Practicing Medicine in Ancient Egypt', *Juniata Voices*, pp. 144-152.

An Approach to Translating *shrt* and *ḏꜣrt*. Compared Methods

Mercè Gaya Montserrat

mgaya001@cofb.cat
University of Barcelona

Abstract: A difficulty we encounter when translating ancient Egyptian medical texts is the identification of drugs. The methods to investigate two of these drugs, *shrt* and *ḏꜣrt,* have points in common and some differences.

shrt:

My doctoral research on the Silphium of Cyrene leads me to conclude that this plant is the *Ferula assafoetida*, white variety. The drug is a fluid that exudes from the plant, used as a solid powder, when dry, or as a fluid, when fresh. Its Egyptian name is not known. The next objective is to identify the silphium-*Ferula assafoetida* with one of the drugs mentioned in the medical papyri.

The information available is:

- The pharmaceutical properties of the silphium.
- The name of the *Ferula assafoetida* in Eastern Mediterranean languages in antiquity, even in Coptic, **ϩⲉⲗⲑⲓⲑ** , a term that can proceed from the Egyptian *shrt.*
- *shrt*, not yet translated, is the drug that has the properties of the silphium and the consonants of **ϩⲉⲗⲑⲓⲑ** . The study of the determinatives of *shrt* is significant.
- The non-medical texts mentioning *shrt* reveal its geographical origin around the area of Cyrene.
- The points mentioned lead to conclude that it could be possible that *shrt* and the silphium- *Ferula assafoetida* were the same drug.

ḏꜣrt:

The method is almost the opposite, because at the starting point what we know is:

- The Egyptian name of the drug and its determinatives that lead to consider *ḏꜣrt* an exudate.
- The information compiled while investigating *shrt.*
- *ḏꜣrt*'s pharmaceutical properties and a mention of its origin from the oasis, lead to identify it with the ammoniac gum, *Dorema ammoniacum,* whose name in Coptic is **ϫⲁⲣϩ**, almost the transliteration of *ḏꜣrt.*

Keywords: Silphium, ammoniac gum, exudate, pharmaceutical properties, determinatives, Coptic.

Introduction:

The translation of the ancient Egyptian medical texts presents some difficulties; among them, the most common is the identification of what we call drugs, ingredients, simples or *materia medica*. For different reasons I came to study two of these drugs, *shrt* and *ḏꜣrt,* and the methods differ according to the different information known at the starting point of the investigation.

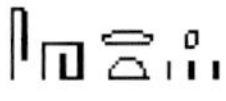 *shrt*

My doctoral research on the today extinct silphium of Cyrene has two objectives:

PHARMACY AND MEDICINE IN ANCIENT EGYPT
(ARCHAEOPRESS 2021): 30–37

First: the study of the silphium of Cyrene, that means the identification of the plant, the compilation of the texts that mention its medical and alimentary properties, geographic localisation, the circumstances of its extinction.

Second: Did the Ancient Egyptians use the silphium of Cyrene? . To answer this question, we must know the translation of the term silphium in Egyptian.

The first objective has several conclusions, some of them are: The silphium of Cyrene is the *Ferula assafoetida,* Umbelliferae, white variety. It is native to Central Asia but also grew in North Libya in antiquity, in an area close to the Greek colony of Cyrene, where the plant had the best properties. It was the most appreciated product of Cyrene and the origin of its wealth; because of that, the silphium plant appears as the symbol of Cyrene on its coins from the sixth to the third century BC.

In Cyrene the whole plant was used thanks to its medical properties, and as food as well. The best drug was the fluid exuding from the root, a gum used as a solid powder, when dry, or as a fluid, when fresh. The juice of silphium was considered the most energetic and light of all the gum-resins, with a great dragging and scratching power, able to drag down a mucus and even a died foetus. Effective antidote, expectorant, carminative, antiseptic, anti-inflammatory, it was a good remedy to heal every part of the body from the hair to the toes. Cyrene exported the dried grains of this exudate specially to Greece, where it was very appreciated as a cure-all medicine and as food flavouring, sold at a high price.

Our next question is to know if it was also exported to Egypt. Because its Egyptian name is not known, the next objective is to identify the silphium-*Ferula assafoetida* with one of the drugs mentioned in the medical papyri.

Information given by some other ancient languages

We know the name of the *Ferula assafoetida* in many languages of the geographical area related with Egypt in antiquity, some of them help to confirm our identification of the silfium with the *Ferula assafoetida*:

Sumerian: aS = *dili* (single); ^{Sam} aS (the single plant). Because the plant was single stemmed.

Assyrian: *Sam xatti re'i* (the shepherd's stick).

Hebrew: *xiltît, Heltita.*

Syrian: *Heltita, agdana, egdana, Halba d-agdana, Halba Qurinaya, ducta* (juice), *ducta qurinayta demen Qurini* (juice of Cyrene), *ducta d-silpion, salpin, silifion, salpin bsc silpiton, opos.*

We also know the Coptic term: **ϩⲉⲗⲑⲓⲑ** (Chassinat, 1921).

A Coptic word starting with a **ϩ** (ϩori) can proceed from an Egyptian term that starts with an S.

Among the drugs starting with an S mentioned in the medical papyri, not yet translated, *shrt* is the one that has the other consonants of **ϩⲉⲗⲑⲓⲑ** .

LVI

(111) ⲟⲩⲕⲟⲗⲗⲓⲟⲛ ⲛ̀ⲧⲉ ⲁⲡⲁ ⲕⲩⲗⲓⲗⲟⲥ ⲡⲥⲟⲫⲟⲥ ⲛ̄ⲁⲣⲭⲏⲁⲧⲣⲟⲥ ⲉⲧⲃⲉ ⲡⲙⲟⲟⲩ ⲙⲛ̄ ⲡⲥⲓⲟⲩ ⲙⲛ̄ ⲡⲙⲟⲩϩⲟⲩ (112) ⲙⲛ̄ ⲡⲉϩⲗⲟⲥⲧⲛ̄ ϩⲛ̄ ⲛ̄ⲃⲁⲗ ⲙⲛ̄ ⲛⲉⲧⲕⲏⲕ ⲁⲩⲧⲟⲕⲓⲙⲁⲍⲉ ⲙ̄ⲙⲟⲥ ϩⲓⲧⲛ̄ ⲟⲩⲛⲟϭ ⲛ̄ⲁⲣⲭⲏⲁ-ⲧⲣⲟⲥ (113) ⲑⲟⲩⲑⲓⲁ ⳨ ⲕ̅ ⲭⲁⲗⲕⲟⲥ ⳨ ⲅ̅ ⲯⲓⲙⲓⲑⲓⲟⲛ ⳨ ⲇ̅ ϩⲉⲗⲟⲓⲑ ⳨ ⲅ̅ ⲭⲁⲣϩ̅ ⲉϥϩⲏⲙ ⳨ ⲕ̅ ⲗⲁⲥ ⲛ̄ⲥⲓⲟⲙ[2] (114) ⳨ ⲕ̅ ⲙⲏⲣϩ̅ ⲁⲛⲇⲣⲁⲛⲏ ⳨ ⲕ̅ ⲟⲡⲓⲟⲛ ⳨ ⲕ̅ ⲗⲓⲃⲁⲛⲟⲥ ⳨ ⲕ̅ ⲟⲟⲟⲥⲃⲱ ⳨ ⲕ̅ ⲕⲟⲙⲉⲟⲥ ⳨ ⲕ̅ (115) ⲉⲕⲉⲓⲛⲉ ⲙ̄ⲙⲟⲥ ⲉϩⲟⲩⲛ ⲛ̄≡ⲟⲥϥ≡ ⲓⲟⲝⲗⲟ ⲁⲗⲩ ⲛ̄ⲕⲉ ⲭⲣⲱ ⲛ̄ϣⲱⲣⲡ ⲙⲛ̄ ⲛ̄ⲣⲟⲩϩⲉ ϣⲁⲩⲗⲟ

(111) Collyre d'apa Cyrille. l'habile archiâtre, pour la cataracte, la taie. l'inflammation, (112) l'obscurcissement des yeux et la ptilose. Il a été expérimenté par un grand archiâtre. (113) Tutie vingt drachmes, cuivre trois drachmes, céruse quatre drachmes, asa fœtida trois drachmes, gomme ammoniaque en morceaux vingt drachmes, os de seiche (114) vingt drachmes, sel andérâny vingt drachmes, opium vingt drachmes. encens vingt drachmes, aloès vingt drachmes, gomme vingt drachmes: (115) mets dans du lait de chamelle: fais-en un collyre; emploie matin et soir. ces maux guériront.

Al-Mashayekh Papyrus, 56. Chassinat, 1921.

In Egyptian texts, *shrt* appears with the determinative  , that we see in terms related to powder or grains, as in 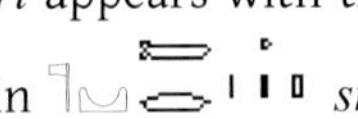 *sntr*, incense, a drug that is also a dry granular form of an exudate, as the silphium is.

shrt also appears (Chassinat, 1933) with the determinative of a jar with handels, Gardiner sign W23, that would indicate the fluid form of the fresh exudate.

Information given by Egyptian medical texts

In the Ancient Egyptian medical texts, the therapeutical properties of *shrt* are some of those of the silphium mentioned in the Greek and Latin texts:

Ebers Papyrus:

To relieve the anus: Eb. 144.
To drain the pathogenic liquid *ꜣꜥꜣ* (àaà) from the body: Eb. 222 = H. 80.
To avoid eyes secretions: Eb. 379.
To eliminate a substance of the head: Eb. 445.
To heal the toes: Eb. 647.

Hearst Papyrus:

To drain the pathogenic liquid *ꜣꜥꜣ* (àaà) from the body: H. 80 = Eb. 222.

Ramesseum Papyrus III A:

To heal the eyes: Ram III A, 24-25.

Medical Book from Crocodilopolis, Vienna Papyrus:

To treat the tumor *ryty:* P. Vindob. D. 6257, IX,7.

Information given by Egyptian non-medical texts

shrt is mentioned in several texts where it is considered a valuable product of foreign precedence, some of them are:

Coffin Text 594 (Faulkner, 1994)

The Akhtoy stela of the Middle Kingdom (Gardiner, 1974)
A geographical inscription at Luxor temple (Kitchen, 1996, KRI II, 621, 3)
An inscription at Karnak temple (Legrain, 1901, Chapel Osiris Unnefer, Nord, 9)
Texts mentioning *shrt* as a substance specifically coming from the western desert:
The Eloquent Peasant R 20 (Le Guilloux, 2002)
The Famine Stela on Sehel Island (Lichtheim, 1980, Sehel Fam. 17)
An inscription at Edfu temple (Chassinat, 1931, Edf. VI, 202,10)

Supported by the information given by the texts, we consider possible that the ancient silphium of Cyrene- *Ferula assafoetida* was the Egyptian *shrt.*

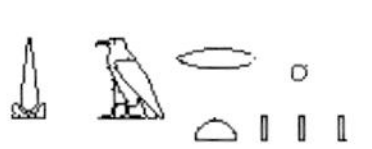 *ḏꜣrt.*

When we study the Egyptian medical texts mentioning *shrt*, it is surprising to see that few remedies include this drug if we compare it with the wide therapeutic use of the silphium described in the Greek texts.

At the same time, we notice that *ḏꜣrt* is extensively employed in Egypt. Among the eight hundred seventy-seven remedies described in the Ebers Papyrus, *ḏꜣrt* is mentioned in one hundred twenty-eight of them, whose therapeutic indications are similar to those of the silphium out of Egypt, for it is prescribed to treat pathologies in all parts of the body (Gaya, 2015); it seems that the Egyptians used *ḏꜣrt* instead of *shrt.*

Scholars differ when translating *ḏꜣrt*, some authors identify it with the carob, *Ceratonia siliqua*, while others propose the colocynth, *Citrullus colocynthis.* The revision of the texts of Dioscorides doesn't evidence a similitude between the pharmaceutical properties of the silphium and those of the carob and the colocynth, while it does with those of the ammoniac gum, the exudate of the *Dorema ammoniacum* Don, a plant that can reach a height of two and a half meters; because of this Dioscorides called it tree (Diosc.3,84). The translation of the term ammoniac gum is not yet attributed to an Egyptian word.

If the ammoniac gum is the most similar drug to the silphium, and we notice the same proximity between *ḏꜣrt* and *shrt*, we ought to verify if the information obtained from the texts allows us to identify *ḏꜣrt* with the ammoniac gum.

If *ḏꜣrt* really was the ammoniac gum, one possible reason for the Egyptians to use it instead of the silphium-*Ferula assafoetida-shrt* could be that *shrt* was a foreign drug, expensive, and perhaps difficult to get, while *ḏꜣrt* was almost local, for it came from the western oases of Egypt that had a fluid trade with the Egyptian towns.

The determinatives

The term *ḏꜣrt* is written followed by different determinatives, ideograms that clarify its meaning and, in some way, some of the properties of the drug, all them fit with the characteristics of an exudate:

A)

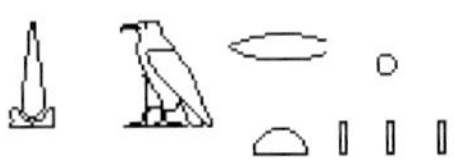

B)

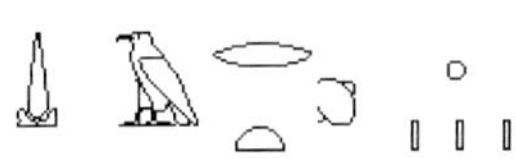

C)

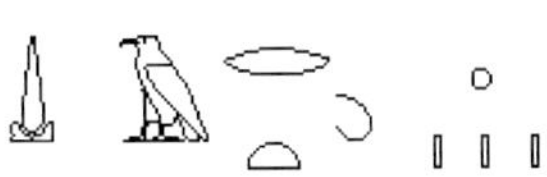

D)

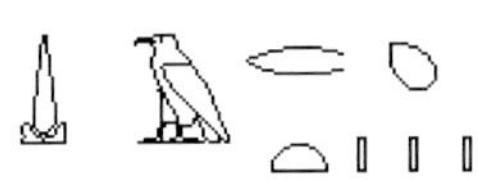

E)

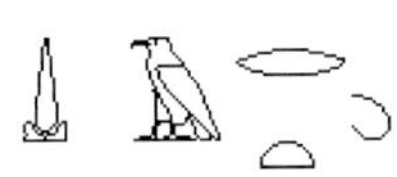

A) Association of the Gardiner signs N33 and Z2. The most used in writing *ḏꜣrt*. As in *shrt* and in *snṯr*, can express powder, grains, solid material in general, as the granular form of a dried fluid.

B) An oval form with two protuberances, Gardiner sign Aa2, determines bodily growths, as an exudate is.

C, D, E) An egg, Gardiner sign H8, expresses filiation. In the case of an exudate, filiation is the relationship with the plant from where it flows. Gardiner also mentions that this sign perhaps derived from an earlier sign for a clod of earth (Gardiner, 1927). The shape of a solidified gum usually is a grain or a clod.

Some texts mention *ḏꜣrt*'s powder (Gaya, 2015) or grains with the determinative of a finger, Gardiner D51, that indicates the action of notching or scratching to obtain the exudate from the plant.

Like other gums, *ḏꜣrt* is soluble in water, for it is given to drink by putting it directly in water.

The text Ebers 212 mentions the origin of *ḏꜣrt* from the oasis. This information is relevant because the name ammoniac gum might have a relationship with the Amun oasis, today Siwa.

Information given by some other ancient languages

The names of the ammoniac gum in Sumerian and Assyrian are unknown.

Persian: *Darukht ushuq, os-chak, kandal.* In south Iran: *yazdé khast*. In Balochistan: *ziarat*.

Syrian: *oshaq*.

There is some resemblance between the phonetics of some of these terms and *ḏ3rt*.

Finally, it is outstanding that the Coptic term **ϫⲁⲣⲧ**, that designs the ammoniac gum (Chassinat, 1921) is the transcription to Coptic of the Egyptian *ḏ3rt*. We pronounce both terms in the same way.

shrt and *ḏ3rt* translations. Compared methods

When studying *shrt* the sequence we follow is:

We are looking for an Egyptian drug to be identified with the silphium- *Ferula assafoetida.*
We know its physical and pharmaceutical properties.
We know its geographical origin from foreign countries located in Asia, and beyond the western desert.
An interesting fact is that we know the Coptic name of the *Ferula assafoetida*: **ϩⲉⲗⲑⲓⲑ** ·
We establish the hypothesis **ϩⲉⲗⲑⲓⲑ** to be the Egyptian *shrt.*
We consider our hypothesis confirmed by:
The study of the determinatives of *shrt.*
The study of the pharmaceutical properties of *shrt.*
The texts mentioning the high value of *shrt.*
The texts mentioning the foreign origin, specially from western countries, of *shrt.*

When studying *ḏ3rt* the sequence we follow is:

We know the term of a drug in Egyptian.

We notice that it was prescribed instead of the silphium-*Ferula assafoetida-shrt* because its pharmaceutical properties are similar.

We establish the hypothesis *ḏ3rt* to be the ammoniac gum.
We consider our hypothesis confirmed by:
The study of the determinatives of *ḏ3rt.*
The study of the physical and pharmaceutical properties of *ḏ3rt.*
The origin of both drugs from the western desert.
The Coptic term, **ϫⲁⲣⲧ**, for the ammoniac gum is the transcription of *ḏ3rt.*

Conclusions

The today extinct silphium of Cyrene was one of the most appreciated drugs in antiquity because of its wide variety of applications in medicine and its alimentary use. We identify the silphium with the *Ferula assafoetida* and with the Egyptian drug *shrt*. In the medical papyri, *ḏ3rt* is prescribed in a great number of remedies with similar indications, this fact let us think that in Egypt *ḏ3rt* replaced the silfium, probably because it was easier to get. The ammoniac gum seems to be the most suitable drug to replace the silfium and to be identified with *ḏ3rt*.

In both cases the conclusions are supported by the information obtained from the texts, that lead us to consider the possibility of the identification of *shrt* with the silfium- *Ferula assafoetida*, and *ḏ3rt* with the ammoniac gum- *Dorema ammoniacum* Don.

Bibliography

Aufrère, S 1983, 'Études de Lexicologie et d'Histoire Naturelle I-III', *Institut Français d'Archéologie Orientale, 83*, Le Caire.

Bardinet, T 1995, *Les Papyrus Médicaux de l'Égypte Pharaonique*, Fayard, Paris.

Barns, JWB 1986, *Five Ramesseum Papyri*, Oxford University Press, Oxford.

Barguet, P 1953, 'La Stèle de la Famine à Sehel', *Bibliothèque d'Étude, 24, Institut Français d'Archéologie Orientale*, Le Caire.

Borger, R 1988, *Assyrisch-Babilonische Zeichenliste*, Neukirchener Verlag, Neukirchen-Vluyn.

Chassinat, É 1931, 'Le Temple d'Edfou, tome 6', *Mémoires Publiées par les Membres de la Mission Archéologique Française au Caire, tome 23, Institut Français d'Archéologie Orientale,* Le Caire.

Chassinat, É 1933, 'Le Temple d'Edfou, tome 8', *Mémoires Publiées par les Membres de la Mission Archéologique Française au Caire, tome 25, Institut Français d'Archéologie Orientale,* Le Caire.

Chassinat, É 1921, 'Un Papyrus Médical Copte', *Mémoires Publiées par les Membres de l'Institut Français d'Archéologie Orientale du Caire*, tome 32, *Institut Français d'Archéologie Orientale,* Le Caire.

Devauchelle, D and Pezin, M 1978, 'Un Papyrus Médical Démotique', *Chronique d'Égypte,* tome 53, no.105, janvier 1978, *Fondation Égyptologique Reine Élisabeth,* Bruxelles.

Dioscorides 1998, *Plantas y Remedios Medicinales. De Materia Medica*, libros I-III, Gredos, Madrid.

Dioscorides 1998, *Plantas y Remedios Medicinales. De Materia Medica*, libros IV-V, Gredos, Madrid.

Ebers, G. (ed) 1987, *Papyros Ebers*, Biblio, Osnabrück.

El-Gammal, SY 1988, 'Spot-Light on Al-Mashayekh Coptic Medical Papyrus (Chassinat Papyrus)', *Hamdard Medicus,* july-sept 1988, vol. 31, no. 3, Hamdard Foundation Press, Karachi.

Faulkner, RO 1994, *The Ancient Egyptian Coffin Texts*, Aris and Phillips, Warminster.

Gardiner, A 1927 rep. 1994, *Egyptian Grammar*, Griffith Institute Ashmolean Museum, Oxford.

Gardiner, A 1974, 'The Tomb of a Much-Travelled Theban Official', *The Journal of Egyptian Archaeology,* vol. IV, part I, january 1917, The Egypt Exploration Fund, London, rep. Oxford University Press, Oxford.

Gaya Montserrat, M 2010, *El Sílfium de Cirene en l'Antiguitat*, Unpublished PhD dissertation, University of Barcelona.

Gaya Montserrat, M 2015, 'La substància djaret', in N Castellano, M Mascort, C Piedrafita and J Vivó (eds). *Ex Aegypto lux et sapientia. Homenatge al professor Josep Padró Parcerisa. Nova Studia Aegyptiaca IX*, pp. 263-272, Universitat de Barcelona, Barcelona.

Jennings, W 1926, *Lexicon to the Syriac New Testament*, Clarendon, Oxford.

Kitchen, KA 1996, *Ramesside Inscriptions Historical and Biographical*, vol. II, BH Blackwell, Oxford.

Le Guilloux, P (dir) 2002, 'Le Conte du Paysan Éloquent', *Cahiers de l'Association d'Égyptologie Isis, no. 2*, Association Isis, Angers.

Legrain, G 1901, 'Le Temple et les Chapelles D'Osiris à Karnak', *Récueil de Travaux Relatifs à la Philologie et à l'Archéologie Égyptiennes et Assyriennes. Vingt-troisième année*, Émile Bouillon, Paris.

Lichtheim, M 1980, *Ancient Egyptian Literature. Volume III: The Late Period*, University of California Press, Berkeley, Los Angeles, London.
Löw, I 1967, *Die Flora der Juden*, vol. III, Georg Olms, Hildesheim.
Parsa, A 1951, *Flore de l'Iran*, vol. I, Danesh, Teheran.
Parsa, A 1948, *Flore de l'Iran*, vol. II, Mazaheri, Teheran.
Reymond, EAE (ed) 1976, *A Medical Book from Crocodilopolis. P. Vindob. D. 6257*, Brüder Hollinek, Wien.
Von Deines, H and Grapow, H 1959, *Wörterbuch der Ägyptischen Drogennamen. Grundriss der Medizin der Alten Ägypter VI*, Akademie, Berlin.
Westendorf, W 1999, *Handbuch der Altägyptischen Medizin*, 1 Band, Brill, Leiden.
Westendorf, W 1999, *Handbuch der Altägyptischen Medizin*, 2 Band, Brill, Leiden.
Wreszinski, W 1913, *Transkription des Papyrus Ebers. Die Medizin der Alten Ägypter*, Band 3, JC Hinrichs, Leipzig.

Palaeopathology of an Antique Population. Kharga Oasis in Ptolemaic And Roman Times

Roger Lichtenberg
lichtenberg_roger@yahoo.fr
UMR 7044 University of Strasbourg

Abstract: About 1500 people living during Ptolemaic-Roman period have been discovered on three sites of Kharga Oasis. R. Lichtenberg, who X-Rayed and studied them, presents the results of his researches, that is a general survey of the health of these people. The most frequent disease was arthritis, possibly related to hard working conditions. Bilharzia, which was common among Egyptian peasants, has been recognized too. Growth arrest lines, which mark generally food insufficiency, are extremely frequent. Some cases are presented: multiple bones myeloma, atheroma, a lot of fractures (skull, femur...), tuberculosis, bilharzia and even typhoid fever and appendicitis. Genetic abnormalities such as achondroplasia, defect of formation of spine, supernumerary toes, have been observed. These results belong to a large corpus of observations which has been mostly obtained by X-Raying on the field.

Keywords: Kharga Oasis, population, palaeopathology, X-Ray, disease, mummy, growth arrest lines

Introduction

This paper concerns a population of almost 1500 persons which were studied between 1982 and 2014. They were discovered on three sites of Kharga Oasis, Dush, Aïn el-Labakha, El-Deir, located from South to North of the oasis (figure 1). Our researches were pursued at Dush (1981-1993) as a mission from IFAO (Dunand *et alii,* 1992, 2005), at Labakha (1994-1997) in collaboration with a team of the SCA (Bahgat Ahmed Ibrahim *et alii,* 2008) and at El-Deir (1998 till 2015) with missions from Strasbourg University (Dunand *et alii* 2010, 2012, 2015, 2017). I was responsible of pathological and radiological studies in the French team directed by Pr Françoise Dunand. Anthropological study of human remains, mummies and skeletons, was made by Pr Jean-Louis Heim, from the National Museum for Natural History, Paris. I remind that pathological and anthropological studies have been pursued for many years by an international team on the population of the neighbor Oasis, Dakhleh, which gives possibilities to compare with our own researches (Dupras *et alii,* 2016, pp. 286-304).

The population of Kharga

Speaking about people from Kharga Oasis I would like to present some faces (figure 2). We were lucky to discover, due to the exceptional dryness of desert, very well-preserved mummies whose faces were extraordinarily expressive.

List of the people which were studied on each site:

- **Dush** (92 tombs): 763 people listed
  357 studied, 64 X-rayed

- **Aïn el-Labakha** (53 tombs): 450 to 500 people

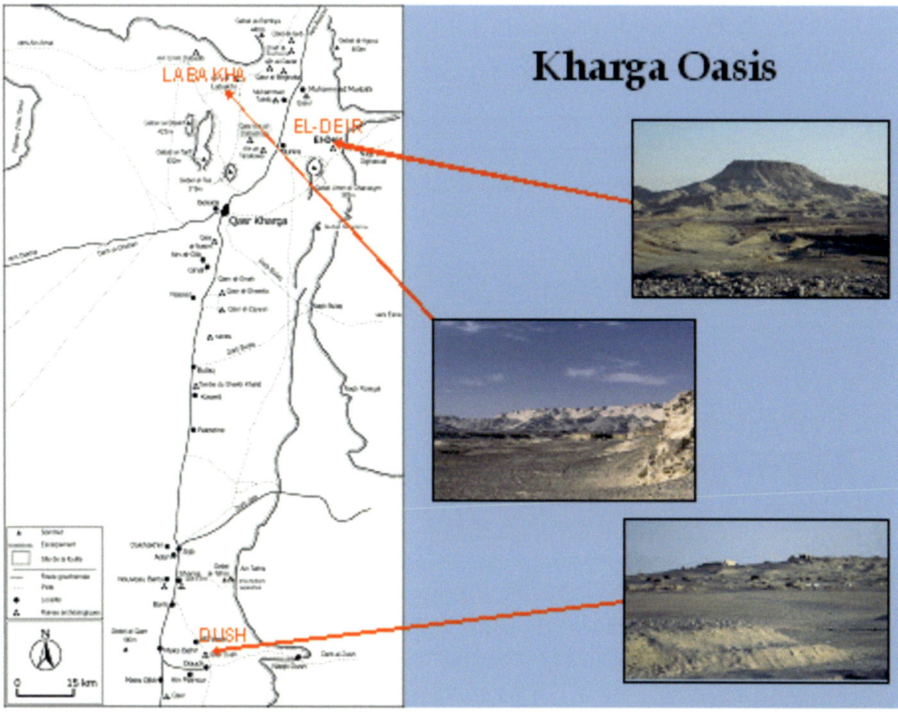

Fig. 1. Explorated sites in Kharga oasis.

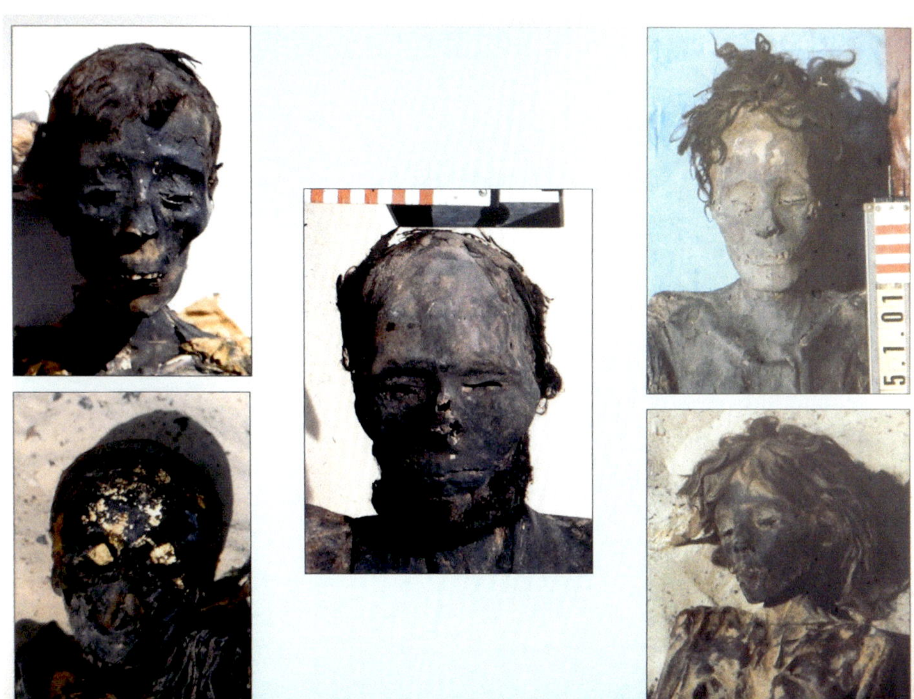

Fig. 2. Faces from Kharga.

67 studied and X-rayed

- **El-Deir** (242 tombs): 1017 people listed
  South (8 tombs): 185 people studied, 19 X-rayed
  North (25 tombs): 210 people studied, 28 X-rayed
  North-East (6 tombs): 34 people, 29 studied, 13 X-rayed
  East (49 tombs): 442 people, 90 studied, 23 X-rayed
  Dogs' hill (4 tombs): 35 people, 22 studied, 3 X-rayed
  West (150 tombs): 111 people, 22 X-rayed.

In this population, there is a large quantity of men, a less important number of women, a lot of children. All ages are present, from immature children to old people over 70. The average age at death was about 32: that is rather important, not very different from the age at death in France around 1850 (about 37).

The number of children is often important, about 20 % at Dush but almost 25 % in the East cemetery at El-Deir. It seems that before 12/18 months they were not mummified; from that age they were often very well preserved, many of them with a characteristic 'swollen' look. We observed a different sex ratio between the West cemetery at El-Deir, which is a Christian cemetery dated fourth-fifth century AD, and the other ones which are 'traditional' as well as much older. Of course, we have not found all the babies who died at birth.

	MEN	WOMEN	CHILDREN	UNSPECIFIED
DUSH	166	117	74	
AÏN el-LABAKHA	32	20	15	
EL-DEIR South	48	34	15	88
North	65	47	44	54
North-East	15	10	1	8
East	81	60	106	179
Dogs' Hill	2	2	1	17
West	41	13	51	6

Tab. 1. Sex ratio.

How to X-Ray mummies on the field

When we discovered the mummies inside their tombs, most of them were rather well preserved, but in bad state, due to the looters or because they were packed without order when tombs were used again for more burials. Before studying mummies, we were obliged to clean them, as they were often encrusted with clay and sand. After that, I was able to perform a clinical exam, to take as many pictures as possible and, at last, to X-Ray the mummies. Of course, each mummy had is own identification sheet where all his characteristics were inscribed.

At Dush, we installed the X-Ray department inside a wooden shed, which was in the same time my bed-room, near the house that IFAO had built for excavations. The mummy was suspended by belts against the wall, so it was easy to perform face and profile incidences by rotating it. The focus distance was 3 meters in order to minimize enlargement of images. The X-Ray cassette was put on a horizontal metallic bar.

At Labakha, it was not possible to install an X-Ray department on the field. The Inspectors of the SCA at Kharga lent me a room inside the *taftish* (Inspectorate of Antiquities) in order to install the X-Ray device and the development laboratory. So, we were obliged to carry the mummies from the site to the town (about 40km).

At El-Deir, we installed the X-Ray department inside a small mudbrick building which had been left by the British Army about 1912, close to the big Roman fortress. There was a closed roofed room where mummies were X-rayed and films developed (figure 3). Mummies waiting for radio or already X-rayed were deposited in an open courtyard (my 'waiting room'). Of course, we were obliged to bring on the field a lot of water and we used a portable generating set.

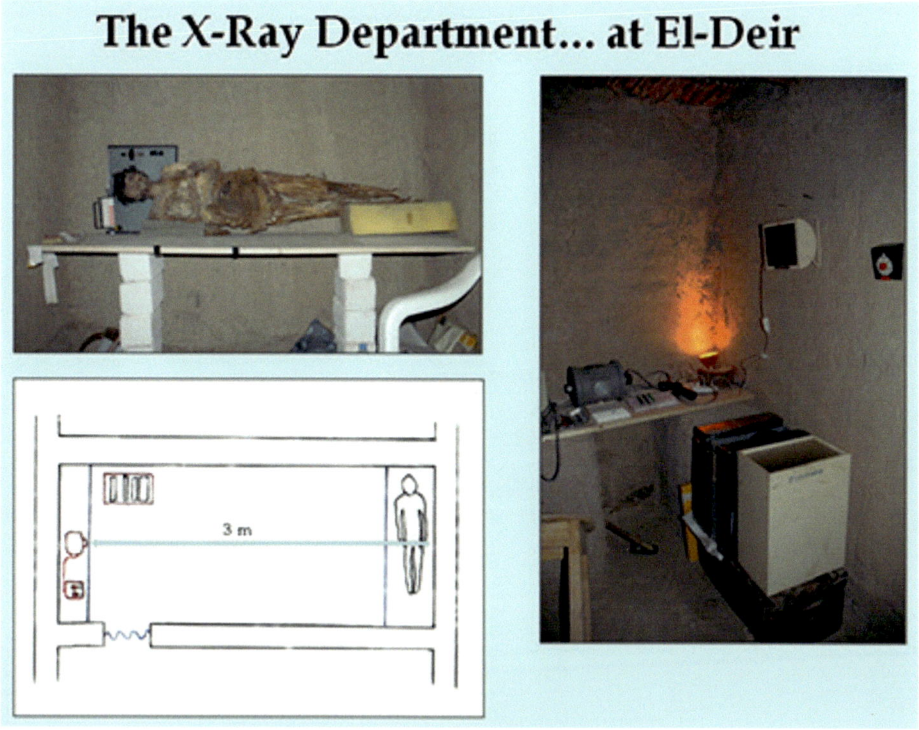

Fig. 3. The X-Ray department at El-Deir.

Now a little bit of medicine

The first remark I must present is: don't trust appearances... Some mummies are good quality outside and inside. Others are misleading, good quality outside, a lot of disconnected bones inside. At Dush, my friend Jean-Louis Heim brought me the apparently well-made mummy of a child (D88.1.1.1): in fact, the X-ray showed the skull of an adult and a jumble of bones with three femurs (figure 4).

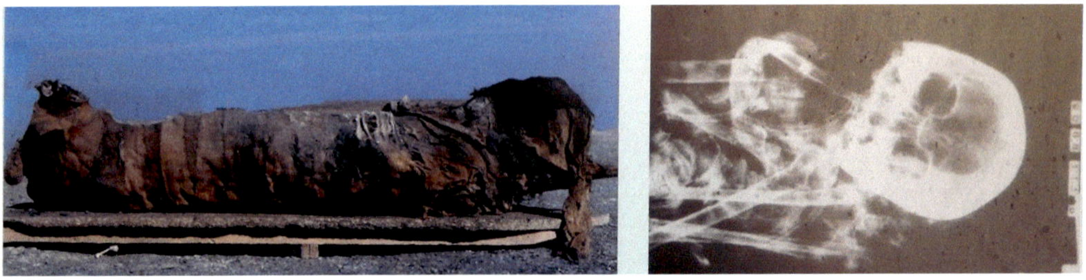

Fig. 4. An apparently well-made mummy, D88.1.1.1.

Of course, the most commonly observed pathology on the three sites consists of bone fractures (figure 5). The skull of the mummy of an adult man from El-Deir (ED.E23.1.2) is badly split on two places, occipito-parietal and left sub-mastoïd. No doubt, it was the result of severe blows hit by saber or battle-axe. It's obviously not so frequent! Another case is more common: after the fracture of femur diaphysis, the man recovered but of course he walked with a limp (ED. S7.1.06).

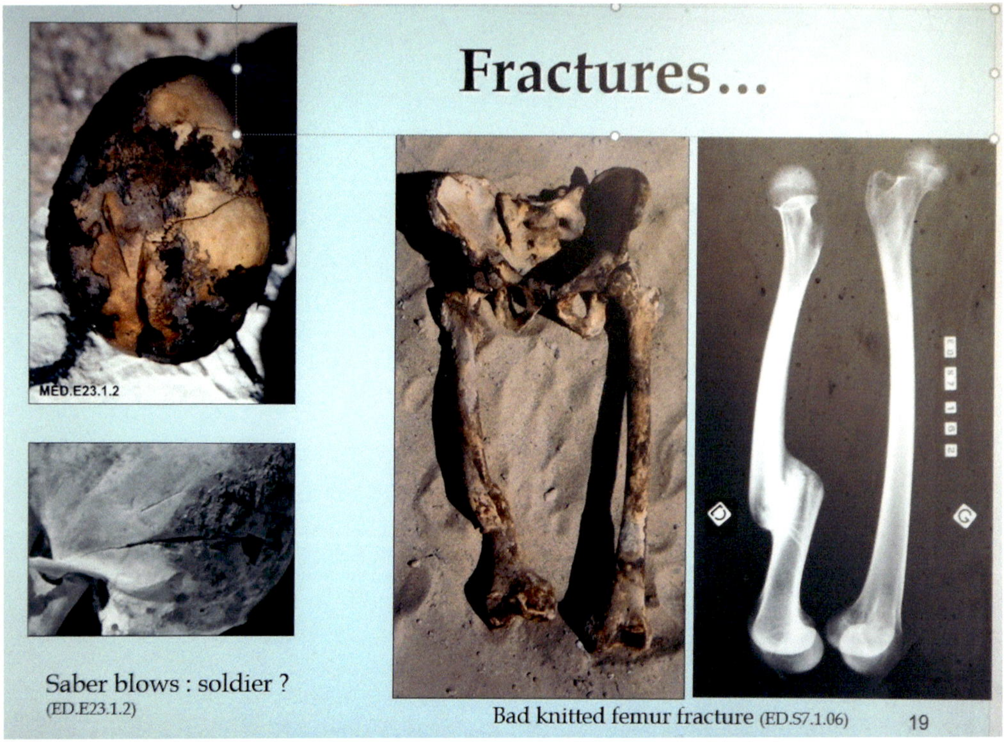

Fig. 5. Skull and femur fractures.

The table 2 shows the most frequent diseases we discovered in the three cemeteries. Arthritis and scoliosis are very common: they were peasants accustomed to hard works. Arthritis was extremely frequent: at Dush, 33 from 53 complete mummies which were X-rayed; a little bit less at Labakha and El-Deir. Arthritis goes rather often with scoliosis: again, at Dush, scoliosis is very present, 43 cases. Moreover, many of these people are decalcified. Bilharzia, a typical disease of peasants working bare feet on irrigated fields, was widespread in Egypt from the end of New Kingdom at least and it was endemic there until very recent times (Sandison and Tapp, 1998, pp. 39-40). However, at Kharga, there were not many cases of bilharzia: we were astonished because we know that irrigation was used in the oases. Other parasitical diseases were discovered like filariasis at Dush (58.2.2.3). Presence of *Taenia* (tapeworm) has been identified on a mummy of the West cemetery at El-Deir (W71.01). Tuberculosis was rare, but it was identified at Labakha, particularly inside one family: three elderly men, between 50 and 60 (AL20.1.02, 05, 08) and a woman aged 30 (AL20.1.03), which were buried in the same tomb 20.

	Arthrosis	Scoliosis	Bilharzia	Tuberculosis	Decalcification
Dush	34/64	45/64	3/64	1/64	9/64
Labakha	24/67	34/67	14/67	8/67	4/67
El-Deir	26/88	24/88	7/88	0/88	2/88

Tab. 2. Pathology at Kharga.

Some special cases

Case 1 (figure 6). An old man, around 70 (AL06.1.17).

He had lost all his teeth, he was rather bald, but his beard and moustache were probably dyed with henna. Calcifications in the rib cage show possibly a parasitic disease. Healed fracture of the 2nd right rib. Arthritis of the dorsal and lumbar vertebrae, with great radius scoliosis. The L4-L5 disk is flat. Arthritis of hips is beginning. The iliac artery present atheroma.

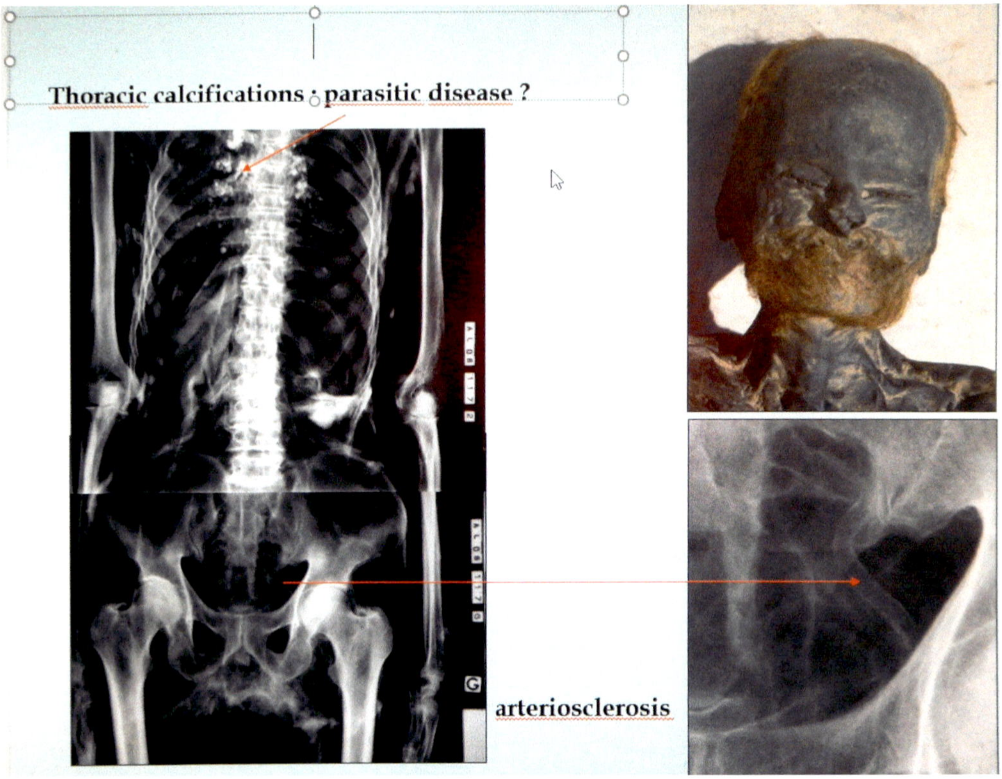

Fig. 6. The mummy AL.06.1.17 (arthritis, atheroma).

Case 2 (figure 7). An adult man (ED.W6.01)

The skull, which has some tufts of brown hairs, presents a lot of almost circular holes. Such lesions are visible too on the spine, the pelvis, mainly the sacrum. No doubt it's a case of multiple myeloma (a kind of malignant tumor developed from bone medulla). To my mind, it's the first time such a disease is found in Ancient Egypt.

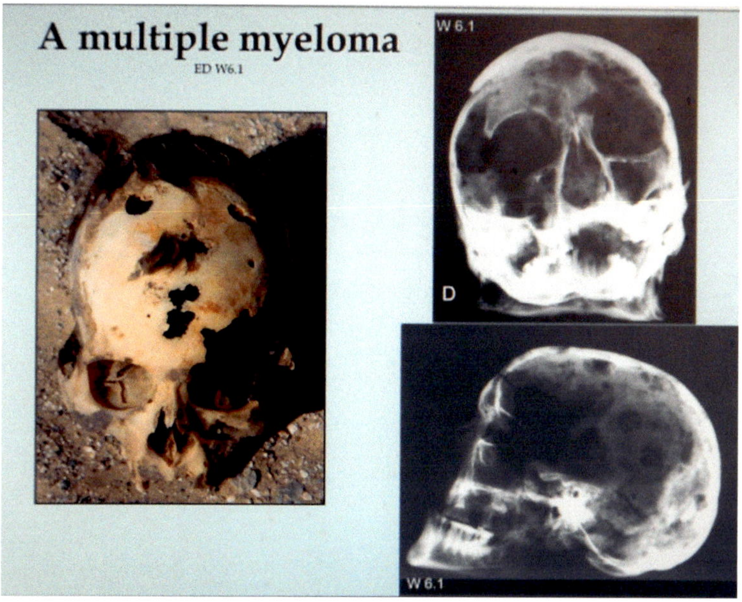

Fig. 7. The skull of the mummy ED.W6.1 (multiple myeloma).

Case 3 (figure 8). A boy (AL.25.1.12)

Here is the mummy of a 12 years old boy who obviously fell down from a high point. The X-rays show a lot of fractures: skull, ribs and left femur, skull fracture causing death, no doubt. Moreover, he had signs of bilharzia on the liver. He presented growth arrest lines too.

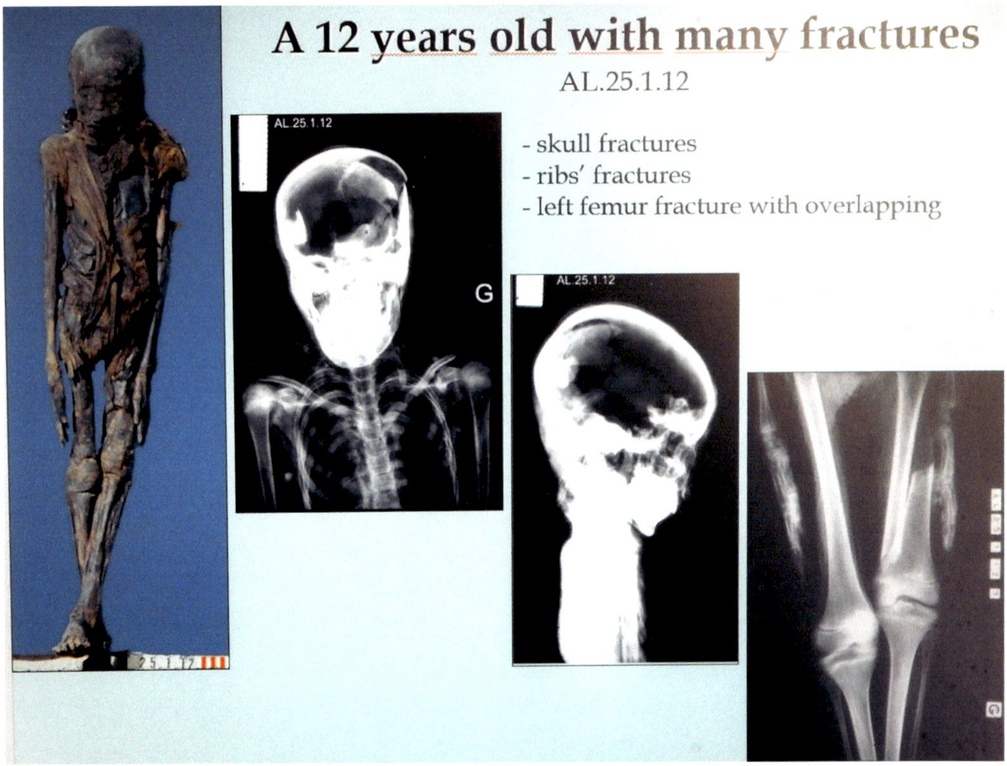

Fig. 8. The mummy AL.25.1.12 (many fractures).

Case 4 (figure 9). An old lady about 60 (D54.1.2.1)

This old woman was rather well preserved, but with her left leg shortened compared with the right one. Obviously, the neck of the femur was fractured; it was confirmed by the X-ray. She is strongly decalcified with a lot of fractures, rachis, pubis, left tibia. There is also atheroma of pelvic vessels.

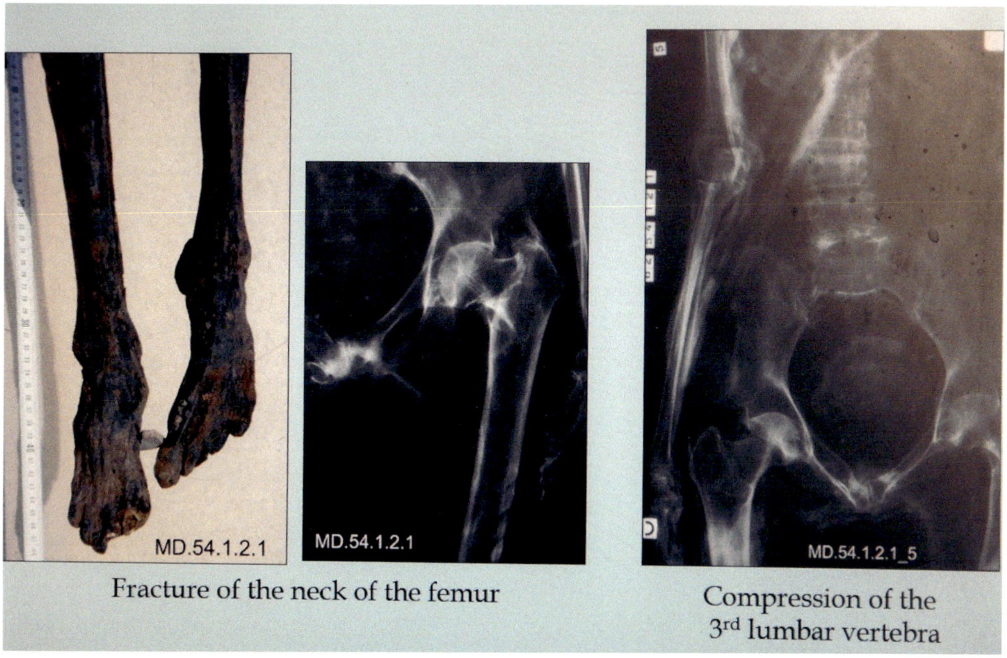

Fig. 9. The mummy D54.1.2.1 (fracture of the neck of the femur).

Case 5 (figure 10). A girl, seven years old (D20.2.1.4)

The mummy is that of a young girl, around seven years. She had a wig. A wig on the head of a young girl? Quite unexpected. Under the wig (made of real hairs), her head was almost bald, with short new hairs beginning to grow. This abnormality can be observed only during one disease: the typhoid fever in its long-lasting form which lead to hair loss.

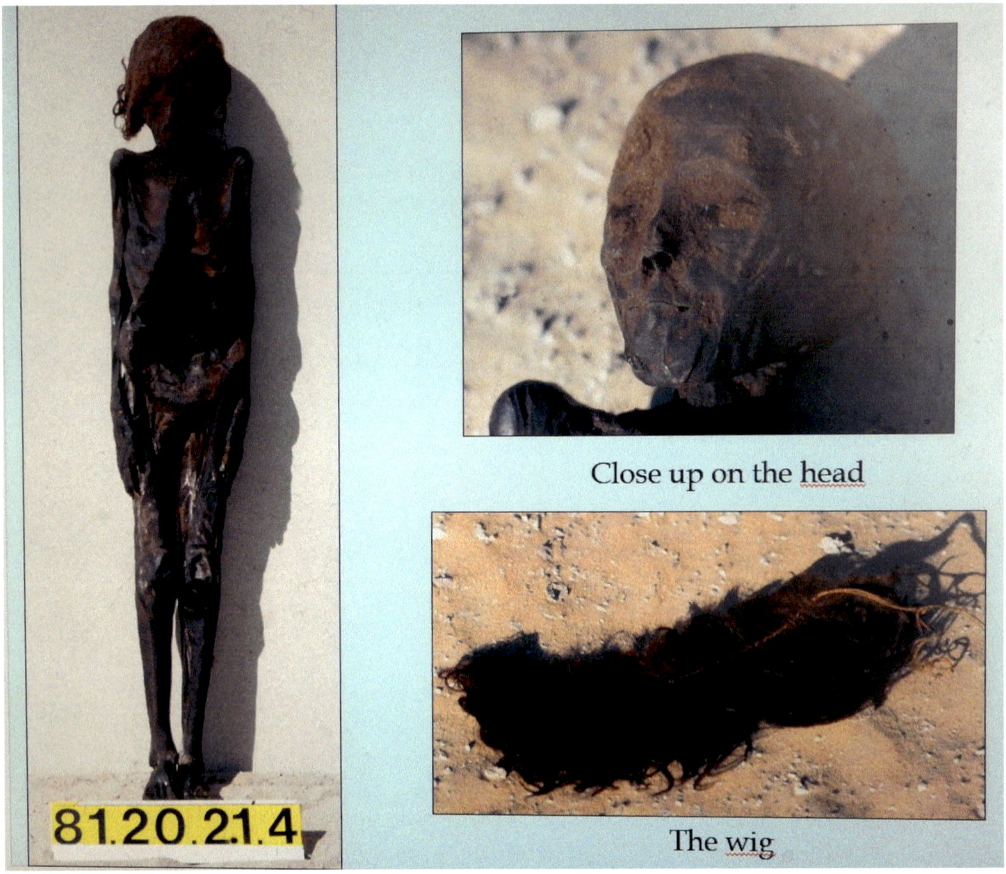

Fig. 10. The mummy D20.2.1.4 (typhoid fever).

Case 6 (figure 11). A boy about five (D92.1.1.1)

Here we don't have any problem about diagnosis. The boy clasps his right hand on his belly at the place of appendix. The X-Ray shows a mass under the hand: no doubt it's an appendicitis with peritonitis. The death of the child must have been horrible.

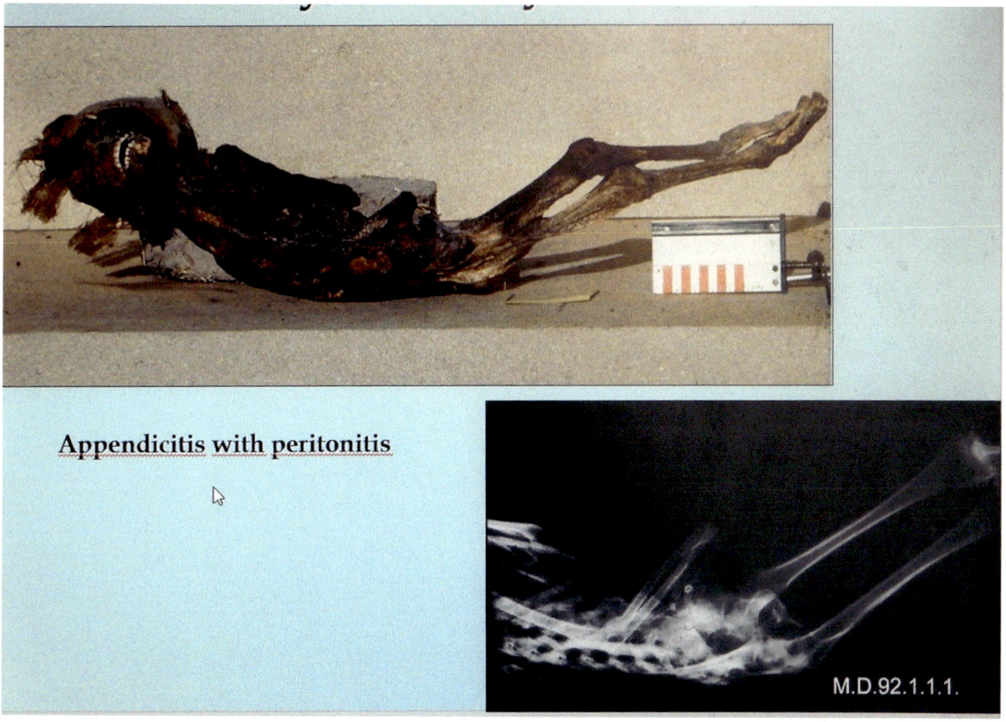

Fig. 11. The mummy D92.1.1.1 (appendicitis, peritonitis).

Case 7 (figure 12). A woman about 40 (AL.25.1.01).

This rather young lady, well preserved, had many problems.

She presents a beginning lumbar arthritis with scoliosis and osteoporosis. The left lung shows calcifications: possibly tuberculosis. The liver and the pelvis show calcifications of bilharzia.

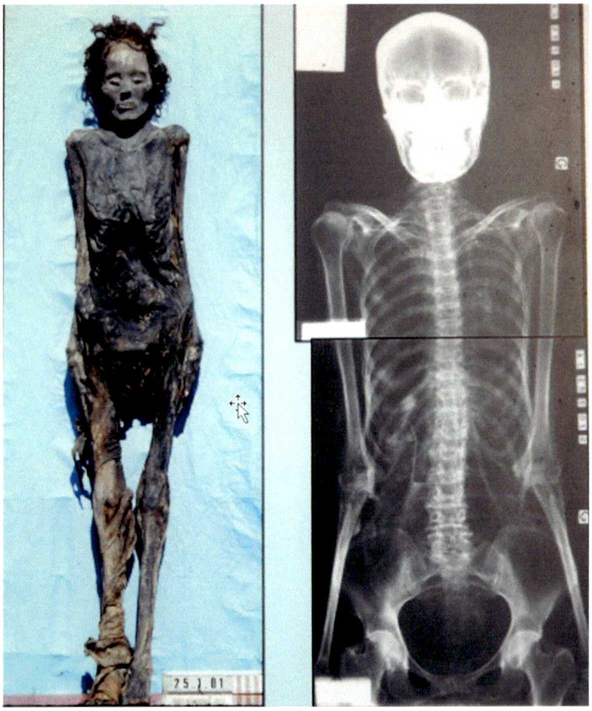

Fig. 12. The mummy AL.25.1.01 (tuberculosis, bilharzia).

The problem of Growth Arrest Lines

(tables 3 to 5)

Using X-ray gives the possibility to search growth arrest lines (or Harris Lines) on the mummies or skeletons. These dense lines appear mainly on the diaphysis of some long bones, particularly on the lower extremity of the tibias, to a lesser degree on the femurs, and more rarely on the humerus. They can be considered as indicating a resumption of growth which occurs after growth arrests caused by rather lengthy illnesses or malnutrition. It's a good indication of an individual's state of health or, more exactly, of his life experience during his period of growth. The ratio of these GAL is very high in Kharga populations: 50 to 60 %.

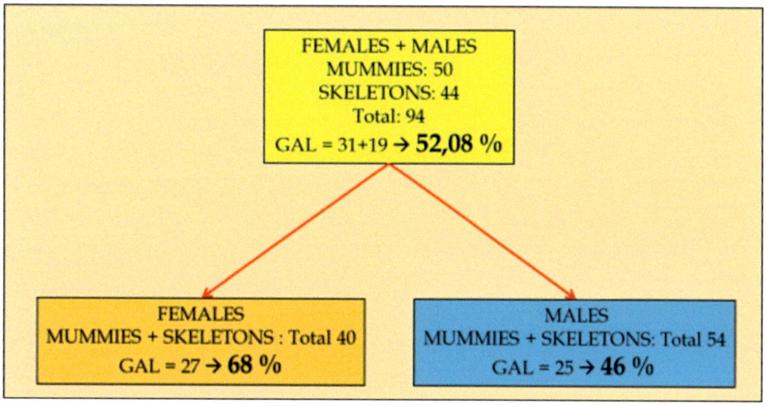

Table 3. Growth arrest lines at Dush.

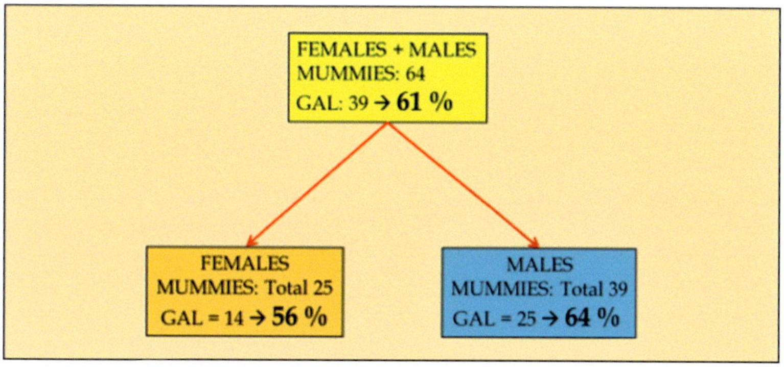

Table 4. Growth arrest lines at Aïn el-Labakha.

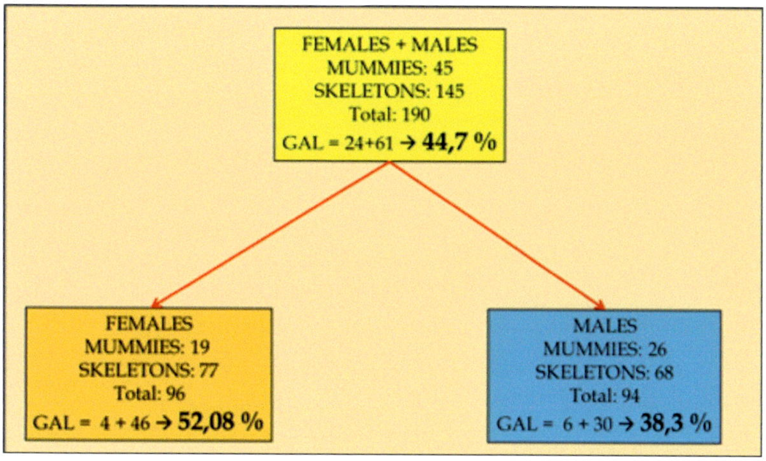

Table 5. Growth arrest lines at El-Deir.

Fifty years ago, mummies from European museums were X-rayed by Dr Gray (Gray, 1966; Gray and Slow, 1968, pp. 28-32; Dawson and Gray, 1968; Raven and Taconis, 2005). They were good quality mummies, belonging to well-to-do people: the GAL rate was only 33 %. The same study was conducted upon royal mummies at Cairo Museum, the first time they were X-rayed; the proportion of GAL was reduced to 5 %, which is not at all surprising: pharaohs could have diseases like common people, but their food was far better (Harris and Weeks, 1973; Harris and Wente, 1980). The proportional presence of these lines within a population reflects the nutritional status of that population. We can say that, generally, at Kharga, people were poorly-fed. At Dush and at El-Deir, the rate of GAL among women is higher than among men. It could be explained by very early pregnancy, breast feeding and food deficiency... When there is shortage of food, men are the first to be served.

Some samples of genetic abnormalities

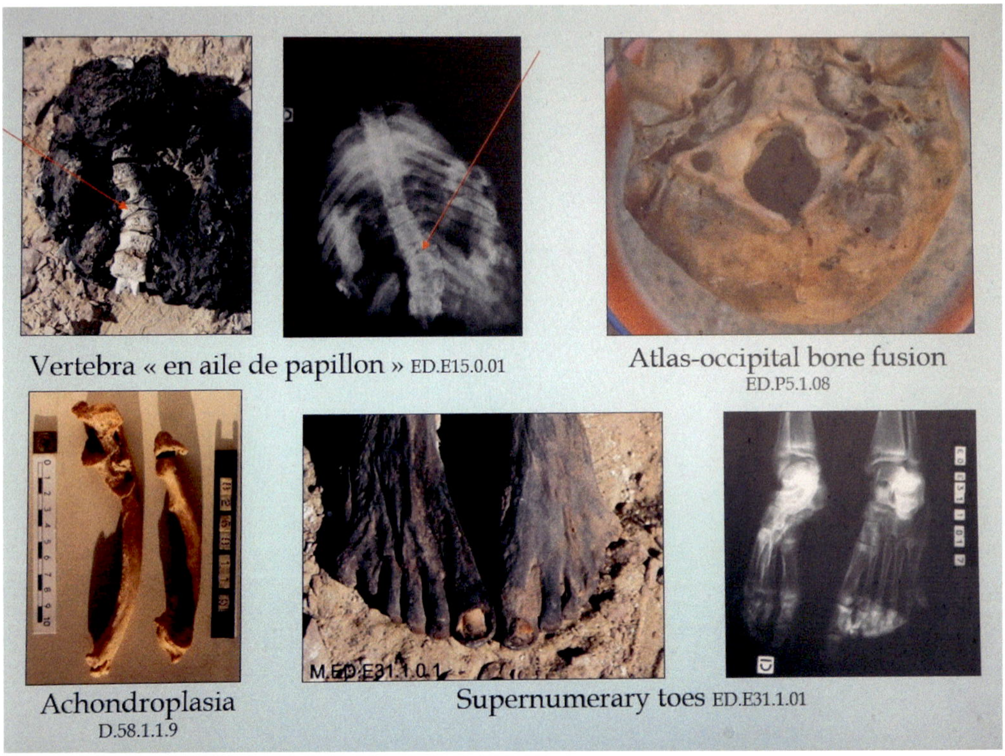

Fig. 13. Genetic abnormalities.

- 13-a and b: mummy ED.E15.0.01, with defect of formation of a thoracic vertebra, French '*vertèbre en aile de papillon*'. The following vertebra is out of shape, responsible of scoliosis.
- 13-c: skull of a grown up woman ED.P5.1.08, with fusion between atlas and occipital bones and spina bifida occulta. This woman had, no doubt, difficulties when moving her head.

- 13-d: skeleton of an old man D58.1.1.9, whose forearm bones present the typical shape of achondroplasia, a genetic disease with causes abnormal growth of upper and lower limbs. He presents too arthritis lesions.
- 13-e and f: a girl (16-18 years) ED.E31.1.01, with supernumerary toes, a very rare case. But one of our workmen told us that it is not rare in the Oasis... We could not know if she had the same abnormality on her hands because they were missing (may be stolen to be used as talisman?).

Conclusion

Till a quite recent time, mummies were studied only in the museums where they were explored by all scientific means. Of course, in museums it is possible to obtain sophisticated results by CT-Scan or other techniques. This paper shows that there is another way to explore mummies. By working on the field, it is possible to survey a whole population. So, we have a complete view of that population, as well common people, farmers and craftsmen, as outstanding persons, civil servants or priests... Inside the museums, we have to deal mainly with well-to-do people, provided with rich coffins and cartonnages.

All figures are from R. Lichtenberg.

Bibliography

Bahgat Ahmed Ibrahim *et alii,* 2008 : Bahgat Ahmed Ibrahim, Dunand, F., Heim J.L., Lichtenberg, R., Magdi Hussein. (2008). *Le matériel archéologique et les restes humains de la nécropole d'Aïn el-Labakha (oasis de Kharga).* Paris: éditions Cybèle.

Dawson and Gray, 1968: Dawson W.R. and Gray P.H.K. (1968). *Mummies and Human Remains.* Catalogue of Egyptian Antiquities in the British Museum 1. London: British Museum Press.

Dunand *et alii,* 1992: Dunand, F., Heim, J.L., Henein, N., Lichtenberg, R. (1992). *La nécropole de Douch (oasis de Kharga). I, Tombes 1 à 72,* DFIFAO 26. Le Caire: IFAO.

Dunand *et alii,* 2005: Dunand, F., Heim, J.L., Henein, N., Lichtenberg, R. (2005). *La nécropole de Douch (oasis de Kharga).II, Tombes 73 à 92,* DFIFAO 45. Le Caire: IFAO.

Dunand *et alii,* 2010: Dunand, F., Heim, J.L., Lichtenberg R., avec la collaboration de Brones, S. et Letellier-Willemin, F. (2010). *El-Deir Nécropoles I. La Nécropole Sud.* Paris: éditions Cybèle.

Dunand *et alii,* 2012: Dunand, F., Heim, J.L., Lichtenberg R., avec la collaboration de Brones, S., Letellier-Willemin, F. et Tallet, G. (2012). *El-Deir Nécropoles II. Les Nécropoles Nord et Nord-Est.* Paris: éditions Cybèle.

Dunand *et alii,* 2015: Dunand, F., Heim, J.L., Lichtenberg R., avec la collaboration de Boutantin, C., Brones, S., Dussarps, L., Letellier-Willemin, F. et Tallet, G. (2015). *El-Deir Nécropoles III. La Nécropole Est et le 'piton aux chiens'.* Paris: éditions Cybèle.

Dunand *et alii,* 2017: Dunand, F., Lichtenberg, R., Callou, C., Letellier-Willemin, F. (2017). *El-Deir Nécropoles IV. Les chiens momifiés d'El-Deir.* Paris: éditions Cybèle.

Dupras *et alii* 2016: 286-304: Dupras T.L., Williams, L.J., Wheeler, S.M. and Sheldrick, P.G. (2016). 'Life and death in the desert: a bioarchaeological study of human remains from the Dakhleh Oasis, Egypt', in Price, C., Forshaw, R., Chamberlain, A. and Nicholson, P. T. (eds.) *Mummies, magic and medicine in ancient Egypt. Multidisciplinary essays for Rosalie David*, pp. 286-304. Manchester: University Press.

Gray 1966: Gray, P.H.K. (1966). *Radiological Aspects of the Mummies of Ancient Egyptians in the Rijksmuseum van Oudheden.* Leiden: Brill.

Gray and Slow 1968: 28-32: Gray, P.H.K. and Slow D. (1968). 'Egyptian Mummies in the City of Liverpool Museum', *Liverpool Museum Bulletin,* 15, pp. 28-32.
Harris and Weeks 1973: Harris, J.E. and Weeks, K.R. (1973). *X-Raying the Pharaohs.* New York: Scribner's.
Harris and Wente 1980: Harris, J.E. and Wente, E.F. (1980). *An X-Ray Atlas of the Royal Mummies.* Chicago: University of Chicago Press.
Raven and Taconis 2005: Raven, M.J. and Taconis, W.K. (2005). *Egyptian Mummies: Radiological Atlas of the Collections in the National Museum of Antiquities in Leiden.* Turnhout: Brepols.
Sandison and Tapp 1998: 39-40: Sandison, A.T. and Tapp, E. (1998). 'Diseases in ancient Egypt', in Cockburn, A., Cockburn, E. and Reyman, Th. A. (eds.). *Mummies, Disease and Ancient Cultures,* pp. 39-40. Cambridge: Cambridge University Press.

A Second Birth to Eternity

Elizabeth Monlouis

emonlouis@orange.fr
Independent researcher

Abstract: Two thousand three hundred and fifty years before our time, Unas passed away. His mummy was placed in his pyramid's chamber. The three portcullises fell, and Unas and the first Pyramid Texts became inaccessible to the world of humans. The hope for a form of survival through a return to the maternal womb probably came into being extremely early in the history of human development. Later, the belief in a life–death–rebirth cycle was carved onto the interior walls of royal pyramids. Indeed, these first texts associate funerary rituals with fundamental knowledge describing the second birth of the Pharaoh. The description of this posthumous pathway incorporates specific medical knowledge, although this is never clearly stated as such. This paper shows that the study and translation of these first Pyramid Texts provide a key interpretative contribution by showing how the rebirth of the sovereign occurs via a real birth, described in all its mechanical aspects. Bearing in mind the initial notion of regressus ad uterum, the phases of giving birth are described via equivalences which, associated with relevant determinatives that will be less specific in the following texts, give shape to hints that make it possible to 'solve the enigma'. The purpose of this work is to outline all the steps of the king's birth, using the translation of the corpus and its localization into the tomb as a basis. The chronological presentation of the phases of birth, as recounted, and the symbolism inside the tomb show how the pyramid becomes like a 'machine' lifting the spirit of the king into the celestial sphere during a perfect description of a 're-birth.'

Keywords: Egyptology; Pyramid Texts; Obstetrics; Egyptian Religion

Introduction

> *'The Egyptians are the first to have exposed the doctrine of the immortality of the soul and the fact that at the moment of the death of the material body, the soul is incarnated in a new body that is ready to be born'. Herodotus*

In 2350 BC, Unas passed away: the pharaoh was mummified and placed in a coffin along the western wall of his pyramid's chamber. The priests recited their litanies, engraved for the first time on the walls surrounding him, and the three portcullises in the gallery were lowered. Unas and the first *Pyramid Texts* became thereafter inaccessible to the world of humans.

The mummified body is supposed to remain unaltered after death, and the texts furthermore explain what happens to the king's spirit: *'Oh Unas, it is not dead that you're going, it is alive that you're going'* (Chamber, South Wall). This sentence referring to the life-death-rebirth cycle belief has since been engraved in hieroglyphs on the inside walls of royal pyramids. The hope for a form of survival through a return to the maternal womb probably came into being extremely early in the history of human development.

Representing the sum of funerary beliefs dating back to Prehistory and associated with the strata of the different eras, the *Pyramid Texts* seek to assure the survival of the deceased king by ejecting his vital principle towards the Polar star. They evoke the different stages of the posthumous journey of the king and his entry into the celestial world.

Both the beginning and ending of the ritual are known: first, the king dies, is mummified and is buried in his coffin, and then, the regenerated king is reborn and acquires immortality during his heavenly ascension. The overall meaning of this ritual is understood, but it is difficult to grasp the meaning of each passage without studying the chronology of the king's displacements and his movements inside the pyramid.

In focusing on the texts in this way, a common thread seems to appear. This systematic approach indicates the presence of recurring themes in every part of this corpus that reveal a hitherto unknown unity. The idea of a moving, active king changing his orientation and the presence of a specific vocabulary becomes understandable only by following a new semantic approach. It is the concordance and chronology of the movements that matters. The king progresses by creeping or thrusting and 'makes his tumble' to put himself upside down. The gods fold him on himself to allow his exit and maintain him during his ascent, 'without ever letting him go'. The pharaoh's positions are particularly detailed on the western gable of the chamber and on the eastern wall of the antechamber.

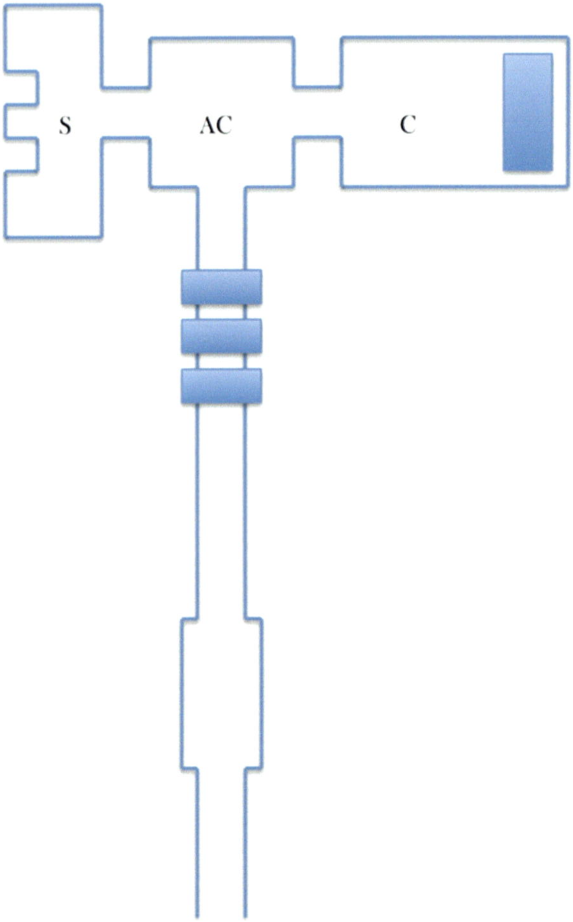

Figure 1 Plan of the Unas pyramid

The king's spirit is propelled through a womb identified with Nut and the sarcophagus which is included in a childbirth process. Hence the Prince's position becomes very significant. Unas is curled up on himself, in the dark, back to the left (the coffin is situated at the far west of the chambers, on the left of the ascending gallery pointed to the North).

The pharaoh must overcome many obstacles to cross the Nun, emerge at the horizon and rise into the sky. His position allows him to present himself head first, while the gathering of the body on itself and the way his head is fixed evoke the position of the baby preparing to leave the womb. This observation leads to a new reading hypothesis: the delivery being described serves as a means of ejection to the sky.

If we consider this together with his position on his side, head facing downwards, we may formulate a new theory according to which the birth is actually described inside the pyramid. Taken from this angle, the stay in the pyramid may be the metaphorical representation of a second birth. The pyramid participates in the ejection of the Prince during the course of a figurative childbirth, repeated over and over in the litanies inscribed on its interior walls, and follows a chronological progression from the chamber to the ascending gallery.

The text uses precise anatomical terms for the designations of the womb, the position and the actions of the associated Prince. Nothing is missing: the modifications of the position of the fetus, a rhythmical movement (the contractions of the uterus) and the risks involved when crossing the cervix and the upper diameter of the pelvis. Consequently, through the texts, the pyramid is depicted as both a pyramid-matrix and a pyramid-machine used to thrust the Pharaoh towards the sky.

The religious context is also strongly present. The actions of the gods that surround the king are very detailed. Their gestures refer to the ethology of the animals that symbolize them, each playing a specific role in the course of the action. They are the actors, the drivers of the pyramid assimilated to the womb, and they regulate its operation. They allow the Prince to rise to the Polar star. They are the guarantors of the success of childbirth, the body of the woman giving birth, midwives, obstetricians, and finally the protectors who repel dangers and support the fetus in its progression.

The pyramid-matrix

The Pharaoh is initially 'locked in darkness', inside a closed uterus that has multiple names. It is called Nut, the maternal womb that allows the king to be reborn. She puts him 'in presentation', protects him from the contractions of Seth, guides him towards the cervix and opens to allow his birth after having transferred her vital movement to him.

> *(171)' the transfer (...) of your animation and the disposition (...) of it inside of you, such as the transfer by Horus of the movement of his mother Isis'. Stanza 595 MN 1640b*

Hathor is the uterine chamber

Hathor is the uterus in the etymological sense of the term (Ḥwt Ḥrw) and known as such, as is revealed by her hieroglyph, a human head with cow ears, topped with two horns that frame a chamber. The comparison with a human uterus highlights a striking similarity: the head forms the uterine body, and the ears and the horns represent the fallopian tubes that we find in the hieroglyph of the '*b3t*'.

> *(574) 'while you are Horus son of Osiris, while you are Unas, the first-born god, son of Hathor'. Stanza 303 WN 466ab*

The amniotic sac is represented by Horus's eye

It is the nourishing element of the Prince because of its capacity for regeneration. It contains an aqueous humour similar to Osiris' serous fluid, which protects the vital energy of the king.

> *(121) ' Osiris-Unas, you have Horus's eye encircling you'. Stanza 128 WN 80c*

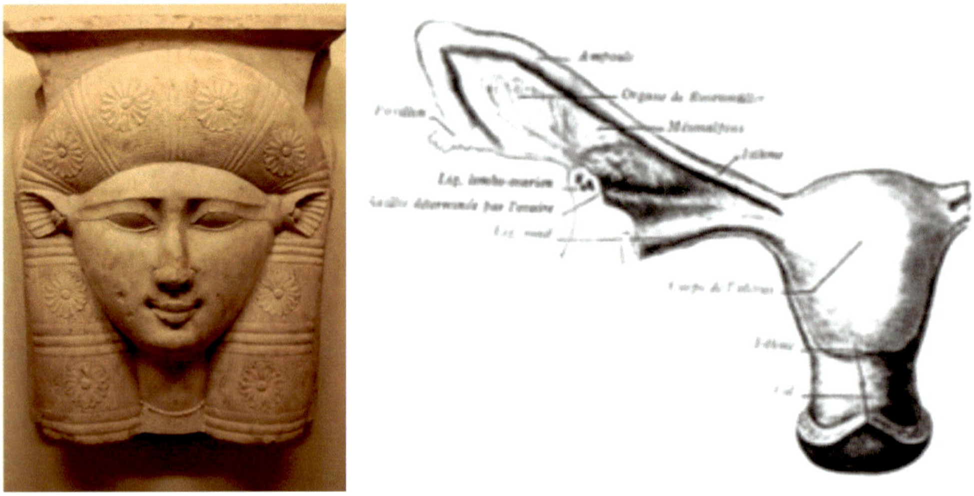

Figure 2 Hathor and the uterus.

(456) 'while Unas is safe in his eye, while Unas's privileged place is his eye, while Unas is resistant thanks to his eye, while Unas is well implanted (at the cervix) thanks to his eye'. Stanza 260W 320ab

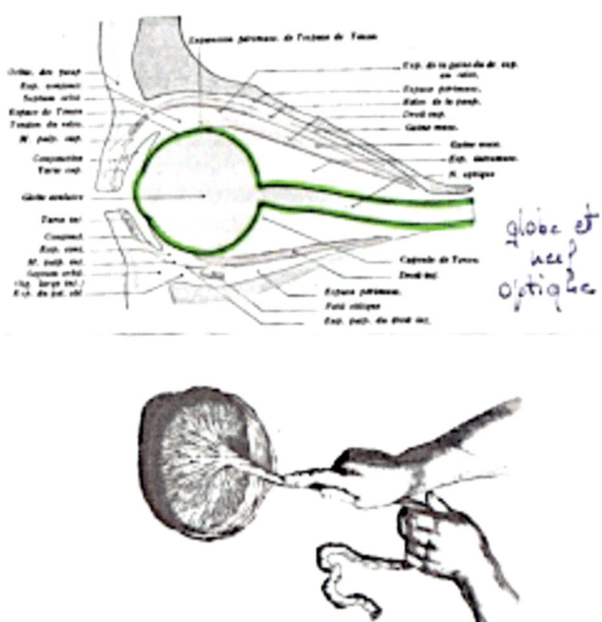

Figure 3 Analogy of shape between the eye and the placenta attached to its cord.

By analogy of shape, the eye of Horus, isolated with its optic nerve, represents the placenta that nourishes the Prince during pregnancy and carries him to term. During the rebirth, it pushes the pharaoh through the cervix, into its channel and introduces him into the flight space.

(95) 'your opening of your channel thanks to the eye of Horus'. Stanza 93WN 63a

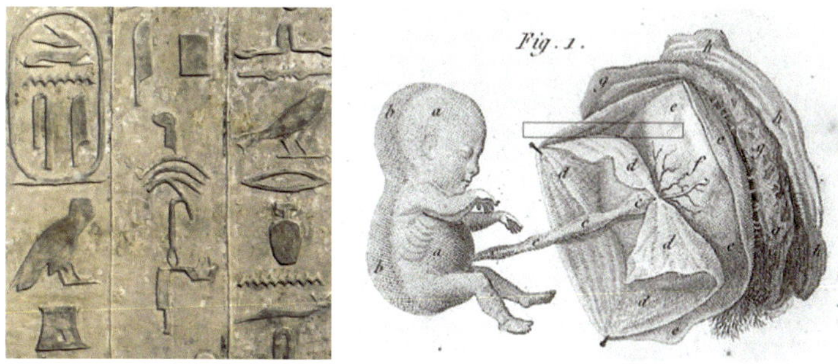

Figure 4 The nourishing membrane, 'the one that unfolds'.

(102) 'Osiris-Unas, here is for you the eye of Horus (for) the widening of his channel (103) Osiris-Unas, here is for you the eye of Horus his engagement from him in your channel'. Stanza 109-110 WN 72c and e

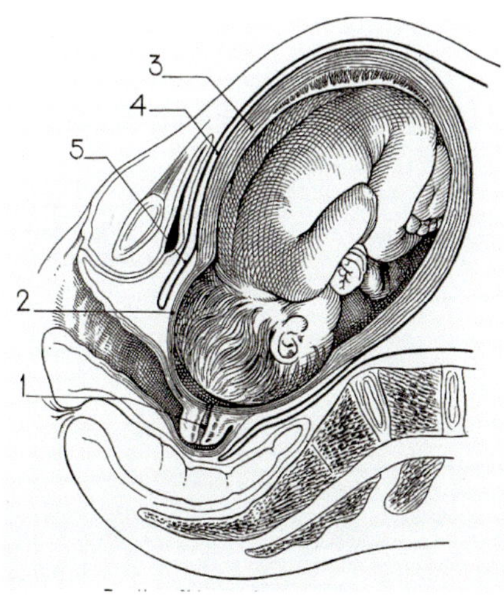

Figure 5 'You will not stay upside down in the dark'.

The hieroglyph of amniotic membranes

It is also the nurturer, the *j3t*, 'the one that is unfolding''. This very explicit anaglyph represents the concentric envelopes of the amniotic sac of the child. The hieroglyph *j3t* is found in this form only in the *Pyramid Texts*. Its role is explained in the following sentence:

(197) 'The nurturer being the one who unfolds, it is she who makes him live, it is she who gives birth '. Stanza 211 WTMN 131de 132a

The 'human' mother does not have a real role in the *Pyramid Texts*. She is present only during the difficult passage through the female pelvis and the locking of the cervix.

The Prince's fetal position

The king is always presented 'on his side' as the fetus at the beginning of childbirth. He is folded on himself, with Isis and Nephthys helping him to tumble thanks to 'the inversion of his two poles', and curled up, buttocks in the air behind the locks of the door to the sky. This position thus recalls both that of the dead and the *regressus ad utero* and that of the unborn child who is 'in presentation', head down and back to the left. It allows him to overcome the obstacles represented by the metaphorical cervix and pelvic bone of the woman giving birth.

Childbirth, the pyramid-machine

The originality of the subject described in the texts engraved inside the Pharaoh's tombs is surprising. In this context, a more religious text is expected. Funeral rites are indeed present, but the main focus is on a second birth, described in its entirety but never formulated explicitly.

As he rests in his chamber, Unas has finished maturing, recovered his vital force and is behind the door of the *akhet*, ready to ascend to the sky. This door represents the cervix that dilates to open the exit canal of the child. The *Pyramid Texts* describe the expulsion of a moving body, the spirit of the king, and depict the process in detail as a birth.

The content of the text, its location in the different chambers of the pyramid and the position of the coffin with respect to the ejection axis to the Polar star (at that time the alpha Draconis, a fixed point in the sky) all contribute to the successful ascent of the Prince's vital principle.

The advance of Pharaoh

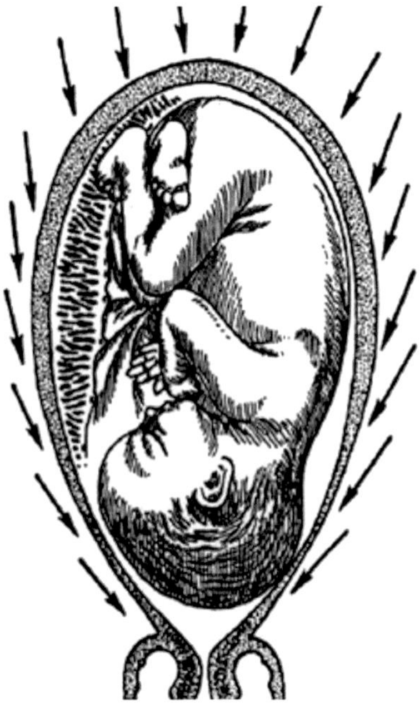

Figure 6 The action of Seth: the contractions.

The contractions called 'waving movement' or 'rhythmic movement' push the Prince forward 'stage by stage' . They are frequently referenced on the southern walls of the chamber and the antechamber (Stanza 258). They start from the bottom of the womb and move towards the cervix, corresponding to a journey from South to North in the pyramid whose gallery is oriented towards the North.

(297) 'Immobilization of you, Unas, undulation of you Unas, your path'. Stanza 224WTMN 218c

(486) 'Perfect coming of the extracted, perfect coming of the leaping, perfect coming of the cleared. Exit of Unas on the thighs of Isis, climbing of this Unas on the thighs of Nephthys'. Stanza 269 WPM 378b 379ab

(524) 'While Unas emerges perfectly thanks to the undulating movement, perfectly mobile'. Stanza 274 WT 414a

28) 'the expulsion of Unas, the perforation thanks to its ıdulation'. Stanza 317W 510b

Animal metaphors : Seth and the contractions

The identification of Seth with the Aardvark is still open to discussion. However, the stanza 277 of the *Pyramid Texts* allows for its identification: 'The sign of Horus being his eye and the sign of Seth being his testicles'. One of the characteristics of the Aardvark is the lack of migration of the testicles that instead remain in the inguinal part. Furthermore, this African mammal has an elongated head, a tubular snout, characteristically large ears and a massive and arched body ending with a pointed and muscular tail.

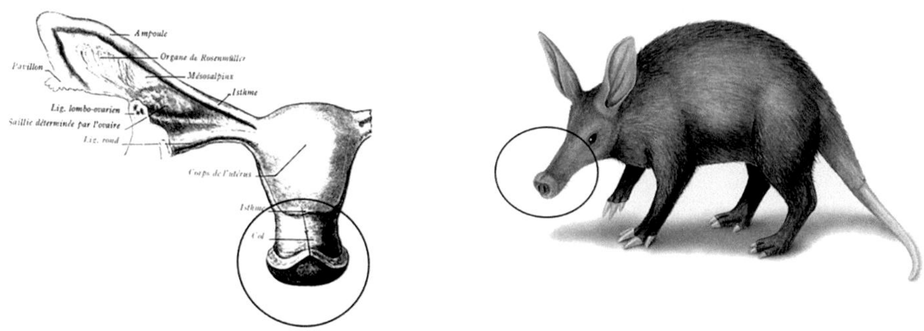

Figure 7 Comparison between the 'muzzle of *tench*' and the snout of the Aardvark.

Seth represents the movement of the contractions. He 'shakes the soil' when he digs deep galleries for 'parasite' animals such as the Lycaon Pictus, referred to as Anubis in our texts.

> *(176) 'Convulsion of the celestial frame, shaking of the ground'. Stanza 472PMN 924a*

As Unas emerges, the contractions of the womb 'spit him' at the opened muzzle of Seth. The cervix of the pregnant uterus is called the 'muzzle of *tench*' in the classical anatomical descriptions and looks like a snout. It is consequently compared to the 'snout of Seth'.

The term *Stš* means 'to spit'. The drool of the Aardvark triggered by Orion and Sothis announces the flood of the Nile, the 'coming of waters' and the flow of amniotic fluid.

> *(462) 'The settlement of Unas on the east side of the Heavenly Residence and the coming to him of the path to the upper [vault]. This Unas is the one who announces the spitting of Seth'. Stanza 261 W 326 abcd*

A perfect staging : The beginning of the timely delivery

The Pharaoh can be likened to several successive gods by analogy of situation. He is Geb when he reaches the cervix and Anubis when he exits. These analogies are numerous on the southern wall and allow us to follow the advance of the king among the gods who surround the cervix. Horus is chosen for his 'high flying' qualities, Thoth-ibis for his long-bent beak and Thoth-moon for his periodicity. Anubis, the wild dog, attacks his prey in the belly. Each element plays a specific role during the birth that seems to derive most often from the behavioural characteristics of its animal totem.

Unas 'tumbles' in the back of the main locks

> *(459) 'The fear of this Unas being to walk in the dark, blind, head down'. Stanza 260W 323a*

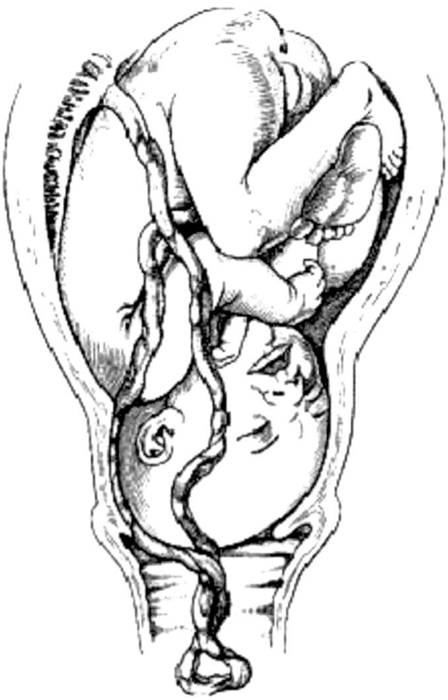

Figure 8 Upside down with his umbilical cord.

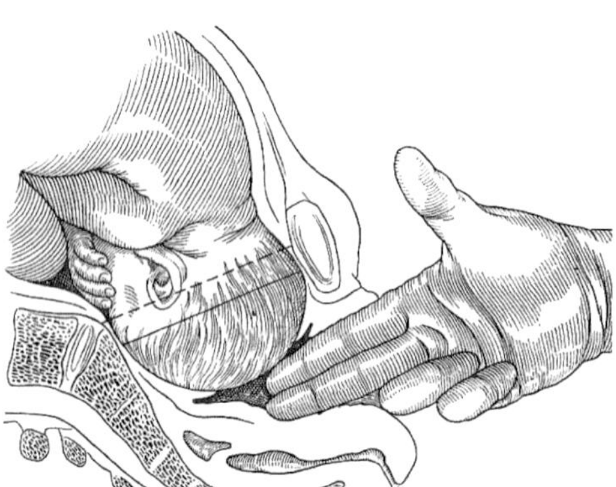

Figure 9 Cervix dilated 'at two fingers of Horus '.

(605) 'Your occiput being outside, (you who are) the one with inverted buttock'. Stanza 551 P 1351b

Dilation of the cervix and formation of the amniotic sac

The 'sliding of the main locks' that accompanies the opening of the womb marks the beginning of childbirth. Unas is aided by the eye of Horus and pushed away by Seth. He must open the doors of the cervix whose opening is measured in 'Horus fingers' and described as either small or large. This vocabulary is relevant since midwives still employ measurements such 'one finger, two fingers' and 'small palm, big palm' in maternity wards. The amniotic sac 'coming out of Anubis' weighs on the cervix accelerating its dilation.

(24) 'The fumigating for you of the end of your channel (and) your spilling of your entire skeleton (25) the end of what affects you'. Stanza 36 W

The 'waters' flow to the cervix. The amniotic sac ultimately becomes visible and palpable by the midwife. Isis and Nephthys check the condition of the fetus at the beginning of the dilation. They are the two 'predators' who keep the Prince in their talons during the childbirth. In the form of two kites, they protect the royal mummy during his journey and put him in the occipital position by securing his head and folding it. They perform 'the lessening of the presentation', then encourage the fetus to exit, summoning him towards the open cervix.

Osiris

Osiris is the agricultural god, representing the Nile and the main nourishing element of Egypt. The Nile is the most common means of travel in a country flooded by the overflowing river for one third of the year. The river is also assimilated with the amniotic fluid that protects the king from uterine contractions during childbirth and whose flow announces the birth.

Osiris is the proto-dead, motionless on his throne, with the mantle that sheathes him revealing the strips of the mummy. He is also the amniotic sac that bathes the fetus in a serous fluid likened to the amniotic liquid and to the aqueous humor of Horus's eye.

> *(188) 'Coming of the Prince to you, master of the celestial setting, coming of the Prince near you, Osiris'. Stanza 477 PMN 964a*

Osiris in his heavenly form is Orion, announcing the coming of Sopdet whose heliacal rising marks the arrival of the flood, the start of a new year and the coming of a new cycle. Unas exits in third place, following Orion and Sopdet on the wave of amniotic fluid likened to a flood.

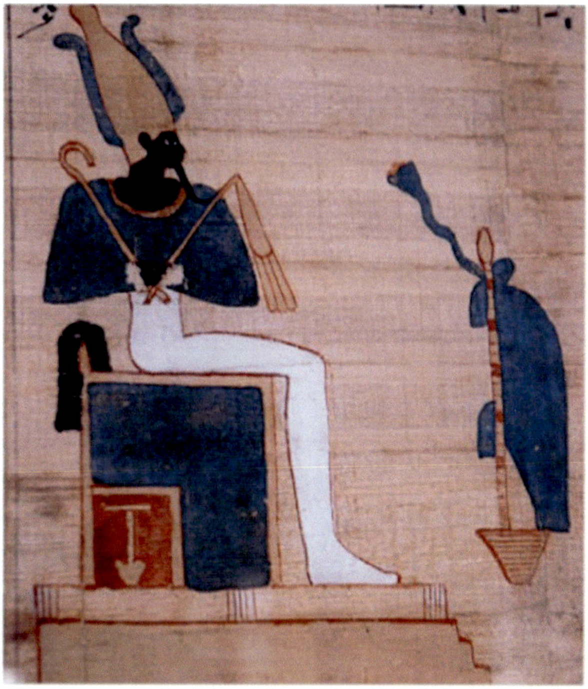

Figure 10 Osiris and his *nebris*.

Perforation of the amniotic sac

In human childbirth, the amniotic membrane often breaks under the pressure of the amniotic fluid and contractions. If not, the midwife scratches the amniotic sac with a fingernail or the tip of an instrument, like Thoth who pierces the pocket with the tip of his wing. The expulsion can begin: the cervix is open and contractions push Unas outwards.

> *(186)'Awakening of the one who opens, raising of (187) Thoth. Awakening of the sleepy, entry into activity of the ones attached to the area of the breach'. Stanza 210 WTMN 126ab*

> *(390) 'The two quills of Horus, (which are) the two wings of Thoth, the two who make this Prince cross, without ever drifting'. Stanza 515 PMN 1176ab*

> *(615) 'As for Thoth, (...) the disposition of the Prince at the tip of your wing, in this other north side of the channel of passages'. Stanza 555 PMN 1377abc*

Before seizing the baby at the exit of the cervix, the midwife can accelerate the dilation of the perineum by fumigating it. The Prince is likewise encouraged to leave the womb by the divine midwives He is still enclosed in his membranes when the amniotic sac breaks and the 'enormous bubbling' begins. He dives in front of Re head first like 'an inverted snake' and exits 'on the tail of the bubbling flood'.

The Role of the midwife

References to 'birth aids' in the *Pyramid Texts* are numerous. They are illustrated by hieroglyphic determinatives that clearly shows the instruments used. The birth of the king must be 'eutocic', that is normal and physiological, because it ensures the immortality of the Pharaoh. If the birth is obstructed, 'against nature', the involvement of the midwife is essential with several possibilities: obstetric maneuvers and the use of extraction tools.

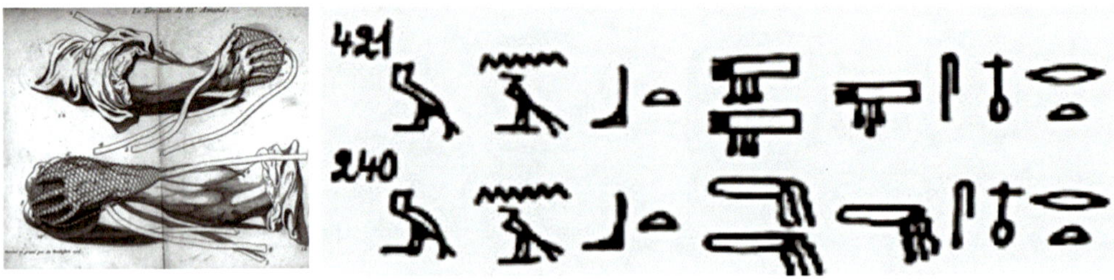

Figure 11 Laces of the midwife 'the one who awaits Unas in the west'.

> *(420)' Here she comes facing you, 'the Western minded', facing you (421) with her prepared curls that allow her reiteration of (my) coming and (my) birth'. Stanza 254WT 282bc*

Mafedet is the genet that steals the eggs in the nests

The goddess Mafedet is often represented in mastabas in the form of a genet in search of young birds in the nest. She is helped by the *shezemet*, 'the one which makes slide', to complete the dilation of the perineum.

> *(312) The emission of your fluid at ground level, your thorax being in the gallery, the fluid spurt, the implantation (313) of the two predators, the completion of your channel by 'that which makes slide', [and] the completion of the channel of 'that which makes slide' (šzmt) by the predator (m3fdt). Stanza 230 W 230abc*

The midwife's instruments

The midwife can avail herself of instruments whose shapes are indicated in the determinatives of Egyptian writing. The links that were used by midwives to fix the baby's limbs are worn around Anubis's neck.

Forceps only appeared in the 16th century. The 'iron hands' designed by Palfyn in 1721 are spoons and branches joined by a link. The forceps of Chamberlen (1733) consists of two crossed branches. Although they do not present forceps per se, the determinatives in the *Pyramid Texts* are nevertheless very evocative.

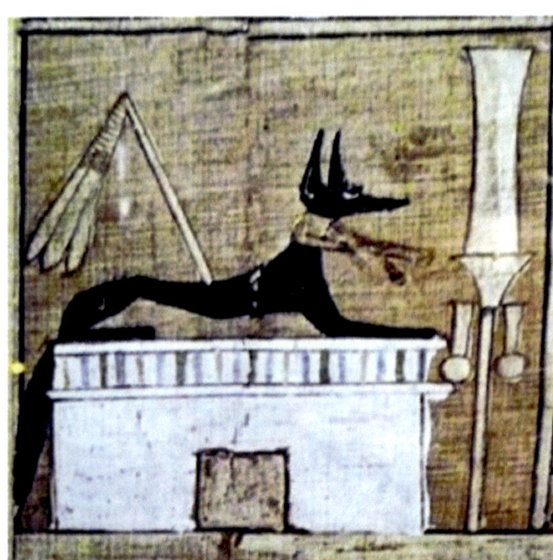

Figure 12 Anubis wears a lace around his neck.

The instruments used are all placed above the baby's head as it comes out. They are clearly named: sticks, dilators and ivory spacers.

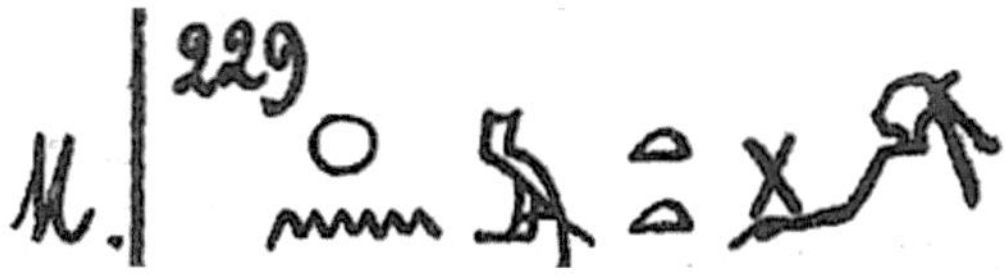

Figure 13 Sticks in the hand of the feeder of Merenre.

In column 229 of the pyramid of Merenre, the determinative of the 'feeder' is a female profile holding in her hand an object that one can interpret as being two crossed sticks. When associated with the representation of the amniotic membranes that follows in column 230, this first drawing suggests the context of obstetrics and birth support. Similarly, in columns 319, 426 and 392, 'two sticks' are implanted to dilate the perineum, 'the channel of Osiris'.

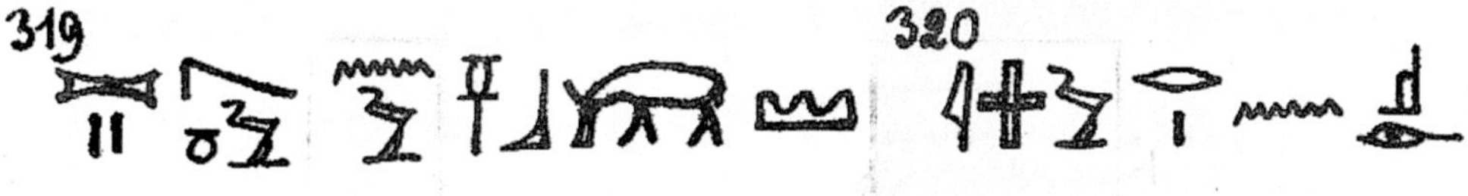

Figure 14 Fixation of the ivory instruments in the channel of Osiris.

> *(319) 'Perfect attachment of ivory instruments (320) attached to the channel of Osiris, straightened by Horus on the spine (vertebra)'. Stanza 230W 234bcW*

> *(392) 'O the ones attached to dilation, (392) O (two) dilators, the stacking for 'the eminent', that is his name'. Stanza 249 W 264a*

Conclusion

The association of death with rebirth is not new. The idea probably appeared extremely early in the history of our species. What makes the *Pyramid Texts* unique is that they are the key to understanding how, through the ages, this concept has gradually made its way from a concrete analogy to a barely recognizable abstraction.

Engraved in a hermetically sealed royal tomb, the first sacred texts of the world combine funerary rituals with fundamental knowledge. The *Pyramid Texts* describe the second birth of the Pharaoh in all its mechanical aspects, employing analogies and relevant determinatives, 'distilled' throughout the texts. The hermetic aspect of this corpus could therefore be due to the fact that although its subject - the rebirth of the king - is globally understandable, the steps of this process are never explicitly presented as those of a birth. The underlying meaning of the text is only revealed in equivalences, which, combined with the determinatives, provide clues that allow us to 'solve the riddle'.

It is not particularly surprising that the scholars of the Old Kingdom deliberately made the choice to inscribe a text describing the king's rebirth, including scientific and even medical terms in a religious building. At that time, architecture, astronomy and the arts were very developed. The faculties of observation required for these fields were equally applied to medicine. This allowed the transformation of the tomb of the king into a 'machine to eject' the spirit of the Pharaoh into the celestial spheres, based on a semantic play.

Associated both to magic (for its incantatory nature) and metaphysical esotericism (for the hidden use of accurate medical knowledge), the description of this posthumous route begins at the top. This journey is found in later funeral texts, but there remains only the idea of a course of obstacles. The primary obstetrical meaning is virtually lost following the *Pyramid Texts*, masked by abstract symbols.

This idea of childbirth seems to be the link between the first funeral rites and those that followed that retain only the symbol of rebirth. The eye of Horus, the nourishing element initially connected to the amniotic sac and its cord, become an amulet with a regenerative capacity: the concrete object is transformed into a symbol and the primary meaning is forgotten. The determinatives of the *Pyramid Texts*, very precise and referring to elements such as the amniotic membrane, do not appear in later texts. They are replaced by simpler determinatives, and the abstract concept they represented disappears. The fetal position so common in those texts is reflected in the position of the conveyor's head, 'he who sees beyond him', as described in the *Book of the Dead*. Thoth, patron of scribes and clerks, records the judgment of the dead and manages the time of rebirth.

However, the obstetrical analogy remains in certain elements. In the New Kingdom, the four chapels of Tutankhamun surround the four sarcophagi, which can be compared to the four layers of the amniotic egg. The Goddess Nut, engraved inside the shelf of the sarcophagi, embodies the pharaoh's mother, instilling life within him.

The *Pyramid Texts* that describe the rebirth of the God-king contain examples of clear, logical thought and are the first medical discourse to somewhat poetically associate mythical time with real time. It seems that this idea in its concrete sense only survives in a symbolic, abstract form in later texts: it would be interesting to explore the topic from this angle. We are in a continuing quest for fertility and the perpetuation of the species by assuring the transmission of life. The Venus callipyges and prehistoric statuettes with marked sexual characteristics proceed from the same idea. Represented as a 'machine to eject', the pyramid represents the means of Pharaoh's heavenly ascension: this is expressed in writing for the first time in the *Pyramid Texts*. These inscriptions are an early example of cosmogony and mythology, presenting an explanation of the world order and cyclical time. The semantic game that transforms the pyramid and the texts that it contains into the first means of ascension for the king makes one of the world's oldest text an extraordinary testament to obstetrics and more generally to the anatomical knowledge of the Egyptians of the Old Kingdom.

Bibliographie

Allen J.P., 1994, *Reading a Pyramid, Hommages à Jean Leclant, BdE* 106/1, IFAO, Le Caire.

Berger C., 1994, *A la quête de nouvelles versions des textes des pyramides, à propos des reines de la fin de l'Ancien Empire,* N°1, pp. 73-80, *Hommages à Jean Leclant*, IFAO, Le Caire.

Frankfort H., 1948 réed.1978, *Kinship and the Gods,* The University of Chicago Press.

Hays H.M., 2012, *The Organization of the Pyramid Texts: Typology and Disposition,* (Volume One) Leiden, E.J.Brill.

Labrousse A., 1996, *L'architecture des pyramides à textes*, t. I, *Saqqarah Nord*, *BdE* 114/1, IFAO, Le Caire.

Labrousse A., 2000, *L'architecture des pyramides à textes*, t. II, *Saqqarah Sud*, *BdE* 131, IFAO, Le Caire.

Midans Reynes B., 2003, *Aux origines de l'Égypte. Du néolithique à l'émergence de l'État*, éd. Fayard, Paris.

Murray M. A. and Dr Seligman, 1911, *Note Upon an Early Standard*, *Man.* Vol 11, pp.165-171.

Experimental Mummification Using Herodotus Description - A 7-Year Longterm Experience of a Human-Sized Animal Model

Andreas G. Nerlich
Andreas.Nerlich@extern.lrz-muenchen.de
Institut für Pathologie, Klinikum Bogenhausen und Schwabing, München Klinik
Andreas Saleh
Institut für Diagnostische und Interventionelle Radiologie, Klinikum Schwabing, München Klinik
Pascale Röcker
Institut für Pathologie, Klinikum Bogenhausen und Schwabing, München Klinik
Heike Freidank
Abteilung Medizinische Mikrobiologie und Technische Hygiene, München Klinik, München
Johannes Fischer, Michael Bock
Klinik für Radiologie – Medizin Physik, Universitätsklinikum Freiburg, Freiburg
Stephanie Panzer
Institut für Radiologie, Berufsgenossenschaftliche Unfallklinik Murnau und PMU Universität Salzburg
Oliver Peschel
Institut für Rechtsmedizin, LMU München, München

Abstract: There exist only rare experimental studies simulating the mummification of human bodies by ancient Egyptian embalming protocols. We used an 88 kg piglet (1,30 m body length) that has a skin surface similar to humans. The corpse was obtained one day after death, cleaned, eviscerated, filled with spices and natron packages and covered with 240 kg natron for 40 days. Thereafter the body was reopened, most packages removed and the surfaces cleaned with wine, the body cavity partly refilled with spices, the surface treated with oils, wax and bitumen and sealed with linen bandages. The body weight was regularly monitored over a period of 7 years.

After 6 years an extensive re-examination (CT, MRI, histology and microbiology) revealed an excellently preserved body that had lost approx. 65% of its weight. The structures of the heart, muscle, skin and soft tissue were well preserved, the body significantly shrunken, but completely intact. Histology and microbiology revealed excellently conserved tissue with anaerobic microbe spores, but only very limited tissue destruction and no significant fungal or parasitic invasion.

Our long-term experiment shows an excellent outcome with near perfect body conservation so that we can confirm Herodotus description providing a successful result.

Keywords: Egyptology; mummies (Egypt); experimental mummification; Herodotus

Introduction

In ancient Egypt the preparation of human bodies to mummies has reached a considerably high level. Following the early dynastic periods where only minor artificial conservation of human corpses was available, the Egyptian culture at its highest levels during the New Kingdom period provided excellent preservation of human bodies. Especially during that period, the most important description comes from Herodotus who described exenteration, cleaning, dehydration, surface-treatment and bandaging of the dead body (Ikram and Dodson, 1998).

Previous experimental studies on this subject have very rarely used human bodies and unfortunately only little data have been published about these experiments. More information is available about other experiments on small animals with considerably different size to humans or animals with a significantly differing body surface (fur or plumage!). Likewise, in 1994, Bob Brier and Ron Wade simulated the embalming of a human corpse according to the Herodotus technique. Since then, this unique experiment has been followed-up and the mummy seems to be existing until today although only scarce information has been published about the experiment (Zimmerman et al., 1998; Wade et al., 2015). Since then, a further human body has been used in an experiment that, however, seems to have been terminated after few months (Vanezis et al., 2011).

In addition, even since as early as 1909 several experiments have used animal models on, however, various animal types: these included chicken, pigeons, mice and dogs. All these animals are very different in size when compared to humans, and the body surface of all those animals in very different to human skin.

In order to more precisely evaluate the effects of the Herodotus method, we selected a pig of human adult size that has comparable dimension, skin surface and tissue composition as an adult human individual. In this report, we describe the results of our model after a 7-years follow-up investigation combining radiological, histological and microbiological analyses after this period of time.

Material and Methods

The experimental setting used an 88 kg piglet (1,30 m body length) that has a skin surface similar to humans. Despite very different anatomy and some difference in the body composition (especially a slightly higher fat content) this model comes close to humans. The body was obtained one day after death, cleaned, eviscerated according to Herodotus description (see Feix, 2001), then filled with various spices and natron packages and covered with a total of 240 kg natron for 40 days. After that period the body was reopened, most packages were removed and the external and internal surfaces were cleaned with wine, the body cavity partly filled with aromatic spices and the body surface treated with a mixture of oils, wax and bitumen and sealed with linen bandages completely in accord to the Herodotus prescriptions. After finishing the manipulations, the object was kept in an open wooden sarcophagus in a room with constantly controlled temperature and moisture that did not exceed 24°C and 45% moisture, resp. The body was kept fully intact and it was only moved out of this setting for regular monitoring the body weight every month/ trimester/ half-year over a period of more than 7 years.

After 6 years an extensive re-examination (CT, MRI, histology and microbiology) was performed. This included a conventional MRI-scan, a whole-body CT-scan, an ultrashort echo-time MRI (TE = 70 µs, TR = 3.5 ms, FA = 16 °, acquisition time = 15 min) (Özen et al., 2015; Fischer *et al.*, 2017) which is necessary under these experimental conditions, due to the weak signal and extremely short T_2* relaxation rates in dehydrated tissues, and finally a sampling procedure. The latter consisted of two 0,8 cm drill biopsies that were taken from the dorsal lower thorax of the body under sterile conditions. Therefore, the surface of the bindings was carefully removed with sterile instruments that were changed repeatedly until the body surface was reached. Then two sterile drills were recovered, one was used for microbiological assays that was further divided into surface and low tissue levels. The second core was carefully rehydrated and fixed in 4-6% formaldehyde, pH 7.4, and prepared for routine histology according to usual protocols.

Results

Preparation of the body and initial manipulations

The preparation of the animal corpse closely followed the descriptions that have been provided by Herodotus (Feix, 2001). This includes the cleaning of the corpse (Fig. 1), the opening of the skull cavity via perforation of the lamina cribrosa of the nasal roof, the incision of the left ventral abdominal wall, removal of the intestine, liver and lungs – while leaving the heart, the kidneys and the inner genital organs in place. Following extensive cleaning of the body cavities, the chest and abdomen were filled with small natron packages, herbs and spices. Subsequently, the treated body was immerged in a bulk of 'natron' that had been prepared before as a 'synthetic natron' in accord with the description of Notman and Aufderheide (1994): sodium carbonate 81%, sodium bicarbonate 10%, sodium chloride 6%, sodium sulfate 3%. The total amount of this synthetic natron comprised 240 kg. The body was completely covered by the natron (Fig. 2).

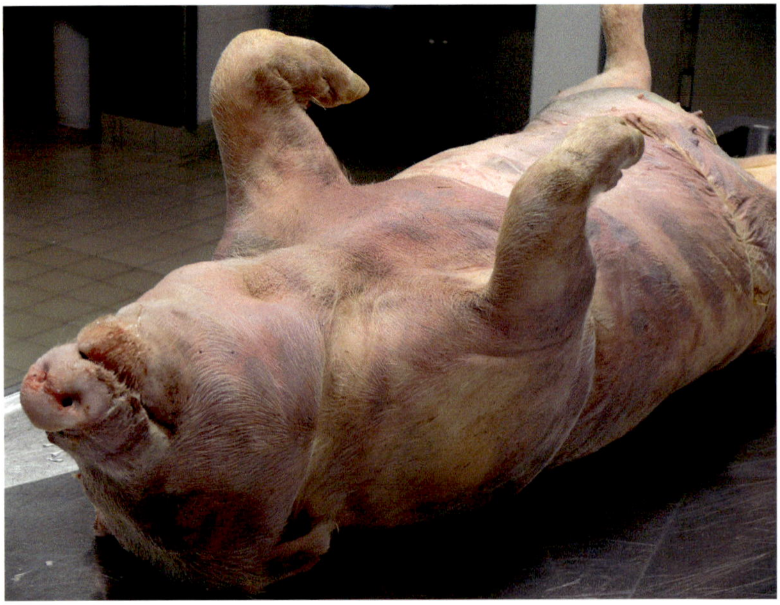

Fig. 1: The animal prior to the experiment

Surprisingly, all manipulations were easy to be executed, with a minimal extent of particular instruments (except for a knife and a special hook for excerebration), nor with special technical skills. The body – with its natron coverage – was kept in a dry place with good ventilation at room temperature (23°C) and moderate air moisture (less than 45%) for forty days.

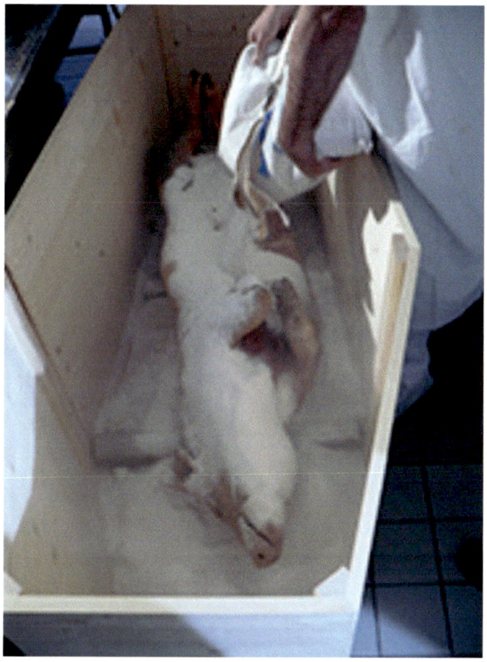

Fig. 2: The body is completely covered by the synthetic natron preparation.

At the beginning of this period, i.e. after few days, occasional small openings were seen in the natron coverage where few dozens of flies obviously paved their way to the surface. Otherwise the natron remained unaltered.

Following the 40-day-period, the natron was completely removed, the body was washed – including a washing step with white wine (12% alcohol w/v) (Fig. 3). The abdominal incision defect was reopened and most of the spices and several natron packages were removed. The abdominal cave was then partly refilled with new spices and herbs in the same mixtures as before. Finally, the complete surface of the body was 'sealed' with a mixture of bitumen (tar) with bee´s wax and oil (Fig. 4) and the body was wrapped in linen bindings (Fig. 5). Ultimately, the corpse was replaced in the empty wooden sacrophagus and kept there under the above indicated storage conditions. The body was only removed from its storage place for repeated weight determination which was determined in the first year approx. all 4 weeks, then every three months and after three years only twice a year. Otherwise the body remained untouched and unopened.

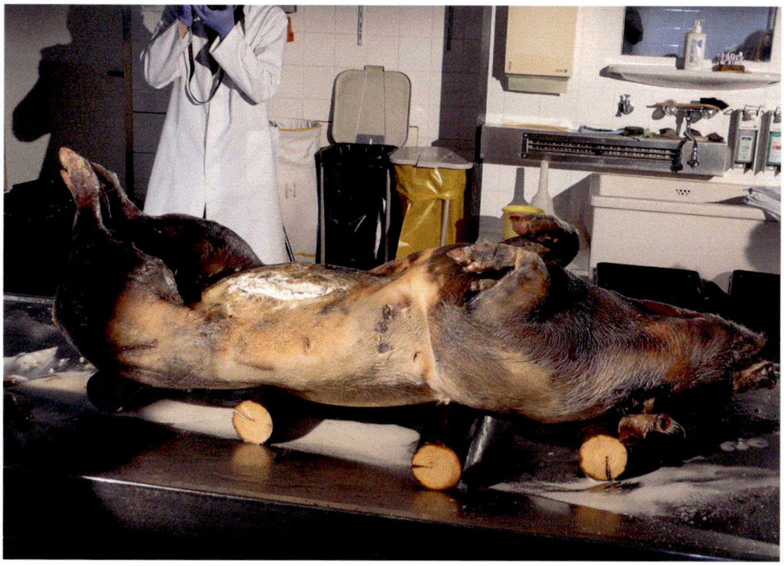

Fig. 3: Following a 40-day dehydration period the body is cleaned. Note the brown coloration of the surface.

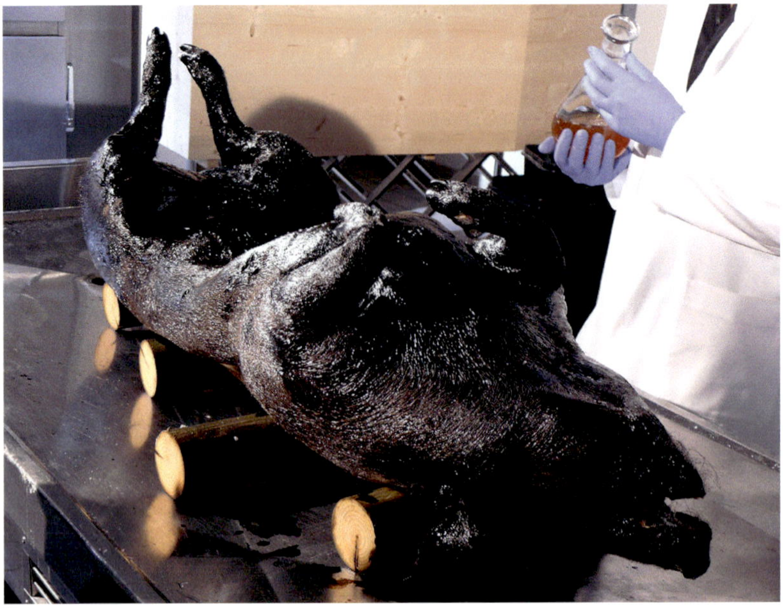

Fig. 4: The subsequent preparation also covers the superficial sealing by a mixture of bitumen, oil and bee´s wax.

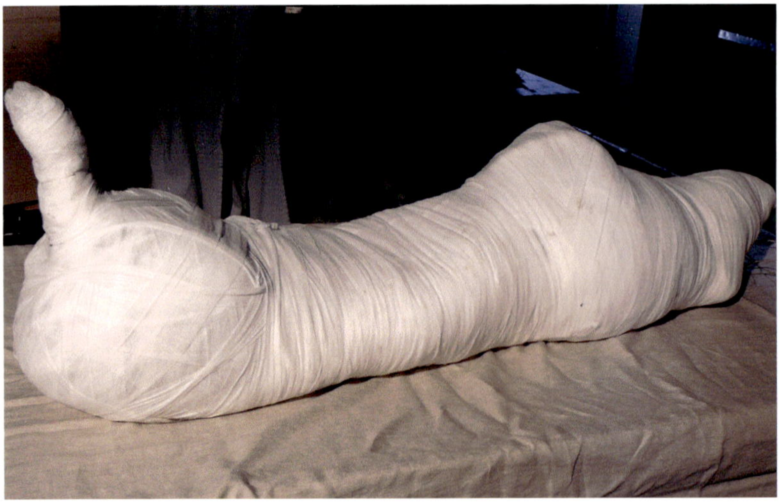

Fig. 5: The body after completion of the embalming procedure.

Development of the body weight

The continuous recording of the body weight revealed a dramatic initial loss of weight of c. 30% within the first 200 days post interventionem, then a more and more flattening of the weight curve reaching the 50% line after c. 650 days and a level of approx. residual 38% of the initial weight after c. 1.600 days. Afterwards the loss of weight was minimal with a calculated loss of c.

200 g weight every half a year (Fig. 6). Finally, after 2.700 days storage the body weight ranged at 32.3 kg which is 36,4% of the initial weight.

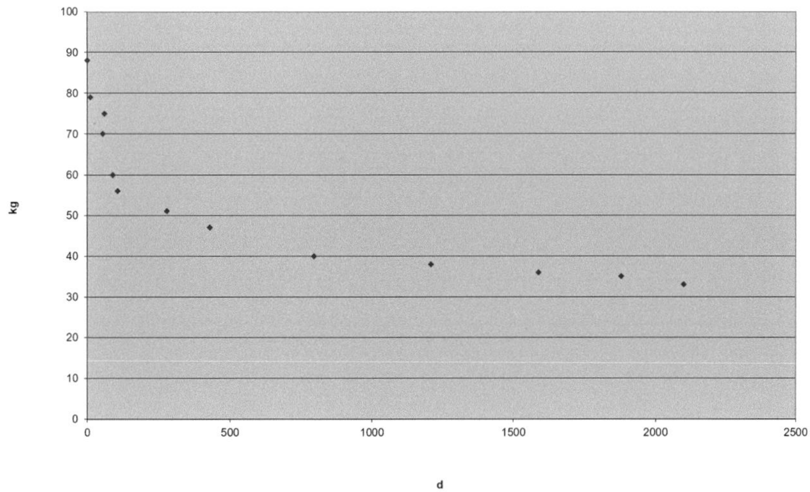

Fig. 6: Weight curve showing the most important data.

Reinvestigation after 6 years – non-invasive techniques

After more approx. 6 years of storage, the body was extensively investigated non-invasively as well finally by a circumscribed removal of tissue biopsies. For non-invasive examination, the body was scanned by routine CT scans that revealed an excellently preserved body with correct anatomical position of all osseous structures, residues of the shrunken heart in-situ, and soft tissue parts of the thoracic and lumbar muscles that showed irregular dehiscence of the muscle bundles with interlacing air filled spaced of unknown origin (Fig. 7).

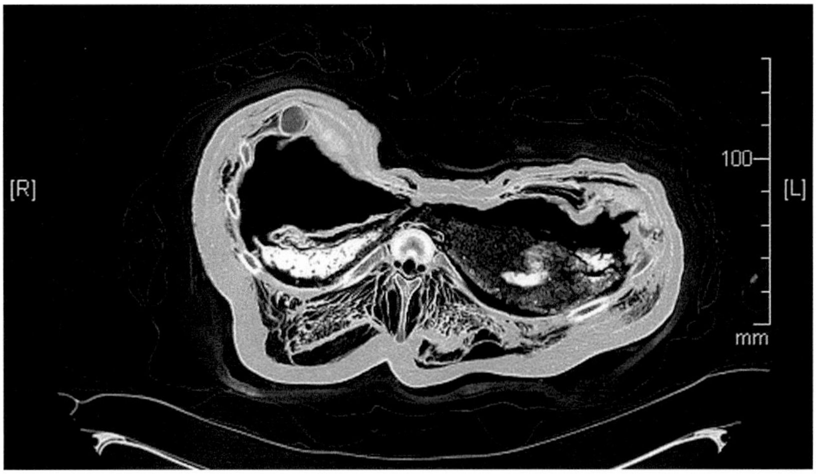

Fig. 7: CT-scan through the abdomen with residues of the natron package fillings. Note the irregular structure of the muscle of the lumbar region.

In order to further evaluate these latter findings, we performed a routine MRI scan which, however, provided only very limited information in T_1- and T_2-weighted images. Further information, however, came from the ultrashort echo-time MRI that had previously been applied to human mummified samples (Özen et al., 2015). Here, the 'residual' water content of the heart muscle provided a layered structure of the muscle (Fig. 8), such as there was evidence for residual water content in the dorsal body wall musculature. T_2* in the heart muscle was found to be in the range of 300 to 500 μs.

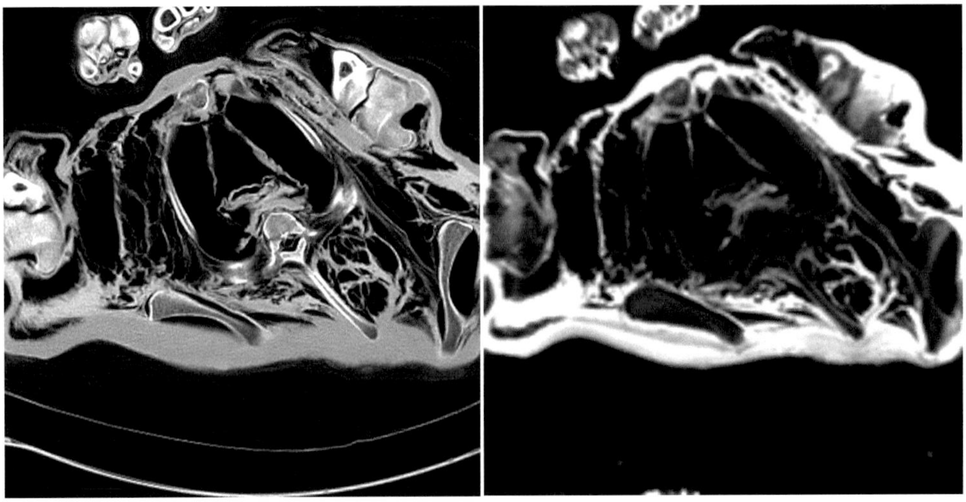

Fig. 8: Ultrashort echo-time MRI scan showing the heart and the soft tissue: though significantly shrunken detailed structures are visible (b). The corresponding CT-scan (a) reveals similar structures although clear differences are seen between both modalities.

Biopsy removal and analysis

In order to further investigate the aforementioned irregular 'air inclusions' in the muscle, we decided to remove two core drill samples from the specimen under sterile conditions. One core was investigated by routine histology. Here, we identified almost intact structures of the superficial epidermis – only affected by a complete loss of cell nuclei – and the dermis, as well as excellently preserved muscle fibers with typical striation and complete conservation of myotube conformations. Between these structures few very small roundish corpuscles were seen that stained positively in May-Grünwald-Giemsa (MGG), but not Periodic-acid-Schiff's stain (PAS). These were attributed to bacterial spores, while fungal spores could be excluded.

The second sample was subjected to microbiological investigation. Direct analyses, PCR-amplification and cultures revealed only bacterial spores, but neither active bacteria, nor fungi. Samples from the surface and the deep soft tissue thereby contained significant levels of spores of Clostridium, most obviously of Cl. haemolyticum species, while the sample part of the musculature additionally contained Bacillus spp.

Discussion

Until today, the excellent conservation of ancient Egyptian bodies remains almost a miracle. Although there exists a wide spectrum of postmortal tissue destruction – mainly due to

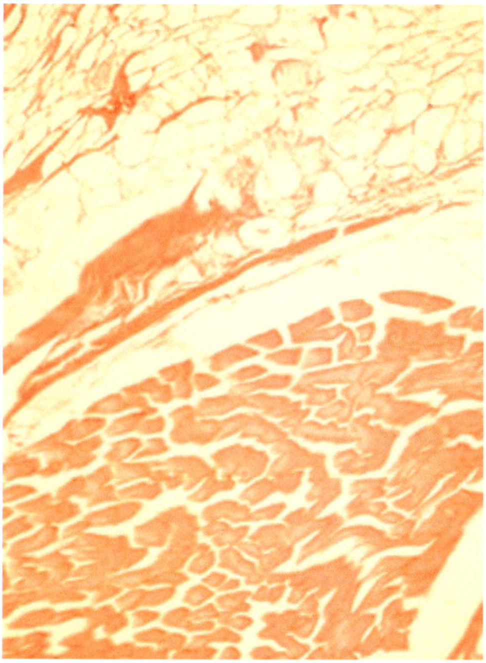

Fig. 9: Histological section through the transition zone of the subcutis and the abdominal wall muscle (H&E).

differences in the storage conditions and the extent of neither anthropo- nor zoogenic interference – one of the most important factors of good tissue preservation is the initial handling during the embalming procedure and the choice of its components.

Although it is now generally accepted that the most important written source on ancient Egyptian human embalming, the description by Herodotus (Feix, 2001), indicates the procedure of cadaver conservation in reality, it is still under debate whether the given time frame, the applied herb and spice mixtures and the surface sealing were effective enough to 'produce' a long-term mummy – with a generally excellent outcome.

Therefore, several researchers tried to simulate the procedure to learn more about the processes of ancient Egyptian embalming (for review see Aufderheide, 2003). As early as 1909 Lucas used 3 chicken that were kept for c. 13 years in soluble natron – at difference to Herodotus description of dry natron. In 1932 Lucas replicated his experiments on pigeons – both experiments with unreported further outcome. Sandison used in 1963 human (amputated) toes, in 1979 Garner performed embalming experiments on laboratory mice for 50 days and in 1985 Notman and Aufderheide used an adult dog that was re-examined after 34 weeks with excellent outcome of the preparation (Notman and Aufderheide, 1995). In the same year Aturaliya (1995) performed experimental embalming on rats.

In 1994 Bob Brier and Ron Wade were the first to use a human cadaver for the simulation of an ancient Egyptian embalming (Zimmerman et al., 1998). This specimen, furtheron called MUMAB, still exists today, i.e. 25 years later. The occasional reports on this experiment provide important insight into the embalming technique and its outcome: accordingly, the procedure was well to be performed, efficient, though costly, and the time frames and manipulations described by Herodotus seem to be successful. Unfortunately, only few and limited reports exist on this experiment – likewise no information is available about the loss of weight over the long time period – a measure that is easily available and significantly indicative. Similarly, only few information has been published on CT-re-examinations, but no further data are available neither on histological nor microbiological examinations or any other additional data.

It took further 17 years that an English group replicated the MUMAB-experiment (Vanezis et al., 2011) – however with a reported follow-up period of only 3 months and unfortunately no information about its further outcome nor on scientifically relevant data. Nevertheless, the 'production' of this second human mummy seems to have been successful as well. Finally, in 2013-2015 the group of Rühli examined two human amputated legs with a broad panel of investigations including CT-, MRI-, microbiological, molecular and histological analyses. These studies provide interesting information in terms of gradual loss of water content, increasing destruction of tissue structures and shrinkage of structures (Panzer et al., 2013; Shved et al., 2014, Papageorgopoulou et al. 2015). Ultimately, Garcia-Jimenez (2018) performed embalming studies on three rabbits.

All these studies provided very valuable insight into different aspects of human embalming. Accordingly, the Herodotus technique seems very plausible. However, several experiments show major limitations: the size of the experimental animals seem to be very different from adult human cadavers, likewise the body surface is very different between humans and animals with furs and feathers, ultimately, the determined parameters and the observation times seem either incomplete or non-plausible.

Our current experiment tried to fill the gap of information – at least in part: we used a model that comes close to adult humans, especially in terms of weight and body surface structure. Thereby, we also circumvented all ethical discussions about the 'use' of a human corpse for the simulation of embalming procedures! Furthermore, we left the embalmed corpse 'untouched' until its first major re-examination – since repeated sampling significantly changes the surface milieu of the body and thereby influences the outcome of the embalming effect.

The present experiment showed a rapid and effective dehydration within the 40-day natron treatment, followed by further loss of weight which was finished after approx. 1.600 days (more than 4 years). Since then, the reduction in water content proceeds only very slightly. It is therefore not surprising that the conventional MRI-analysis after 6 years did not provide major diagnostic information. However, the ultrashort echo-time MRI, using long acquisition times due to the low abundance of protons, allows imaging of dry or solid materials and revealed well preserved fine structures in the remaining organs, such as the heart muscle. The general structures of skin and soft tissue also were very well preserved and revealed detailed fine structures.

CT and experimental MRI further indicated irregular 'destruction' of the muscle, particularly in the dorsal abdominal wall. The 'defects' appeared to be air-containing. As it was unclear whether these alterations may reveal decay or not, we decided to take biopsies from such a region. Surprisingly, the histological tissue structures were excellently preserved and only minimal destruction was evident. In parallel, there was no evidence for active bacterial invasion. Even more surprisingly the excellently conserved tissue contained only anaerobic microbe spores and occasional Bacillus Spp.

Our long-term experiment shows an excellent outcome with perfect body conservation so that we can confirm Herodotus description providing a successful result. Since the experiment is still ongoing, we are curious about the further progress of 'our' mummy.

References

Aturaliya, S., Wallgren, J., Aufderheide, A.C. 1984. Studies in human taphonomy. I. an experimental animal model. Actas I Congresso Mummy Studies, Tenerife, pp. 803-812.

Aufderheide, A.C. 2003. The Scientific Study of Mummies, Cambridge.

Fischer, J., Özen, A.C., Kurzhunov, D., Reisert, M., Tesfai, A., Rühli, F., Ludwig, U., Bock, M. 2017. Cross-modality MR image reconstruction: CT-constrained anisotropic diffusion to preserve edge information in MRI of an ancient mummified hand. ISMRM 2017.

García-Jiménez, L., 2018. Application of oils and resins during the process of mummification: experimental analysis and study problems. 3rd International Conference on Pharmacy and Medicine in Ancient Egypt, Barcelona p. 37 (Abstract).

Garner, R. 1979. Experimental mummification. in: David AR, The Manchester Mummy Project, pp. 19 – 24.

Feix, J. (Hrsg.) 2001. Herodot: Historien. Buch II. Reihe Tusculum. Artemis and Winkler/Patmos Verlag, Düsseldorf.

Ikram, S., Dodson, A. 1998. The Mummy in Ancient Egypt: Equipping the Dead for Eternity. Thames and Hudson, London.

Micozzi, M.S., Sledzik, P.S. 1984. Postmortem preservation of human remains: natural and technical process. Actas I Congresso Mummy Studies, Tenerife, pp. 759 -764.

Notman, D.N.H., Aufderheide, A.C. 1984. Experimental mummification and computed imaging. Actas I Congresso Mummy Studies, Tenerife, pp. 821-828.

Özen, A.C., Ludwig, U., Öhrström, L.M., Rühli, F., Bock, M. 2015. Comparison of ultrashort echo time sequences for MRI of an ancient mummified human hand. Magnetic Resonance in Medicine 75, 701-708.

Panzer, S., Borumandi, F., Wanek, J., Papageorgopoulou, C., Shved, N., Colacicco, G., Rühli, F.J. 2013. Modeling ancient Egyptian embalming: radiological assessment of experimentally mummified human tissue by CT and MRI. Skeletal Radiol 42: 1527-1535.

Papageorgopoulou, C., Shved, N., Wanek, J., Rühli, F.J. 2015. Modeling ancient Egyptian mummification on fresh human tissue: macroscopic and histological aspects. Anat Rec 298, 974-987.

Shved, N., Haas, C., Papageorgopoulou, C., Akguel, G., Paulsen, K., Bouwman, A., Warinner, C., Rühli, F.J. 2014. Post mortem DNA degradation of human tissue experimentally mummified in salt. PLOSOne 9, e110753, 1-10.

Vanezis, P., Buckley, S., Fletcher, J., Coe, M. 2011. Positive reaction to mummy show. The Scarborough News, 26. 10. 2011.

Wade, A.D., Beckett, R.G., Conlogue, G.J., Gonzalez, R., Wade, R., Brier, B. 2015. MUMAB: a conversation with the past. Anat Rec 298, 954-973.

Zimmermann, M., Brier, B., Wade, R.S. 1998. Twentieth-century replication of an Egyptian mummy: implications for paleopathology. Am J Phys Anthropol 107: 417-420.

A Case for Disease Control in Captured Birds Using Hyena Saliva?

Rosalind Park

rosalind.park@shaw.ca
Independent scholar

Abstract: This article takes a fresh look at the portrayal of hyenas during the Old Kingdom, particularly the well-known scenes in daily life tomb art, which appear to depict the force-feeding of hyenas. Typically, this occurs near a poultry yard where ducks and geese are also being force-fed. (Ikram 2001, Table 2) identifies four tombs with images depicting hyenas being force-fed. Since then a report on a further tomb has been published (Kanawati 2006). Collectively, these scenes show tied-up hyenas seemingly being force-fed pellets of bread. Harpur and Scremin (2006, p. 405) suggest that the scene depicted in the mastaba of Kagemni shows a nearby shelf of prepared poultry, within the hyena's line of sight, presumably to encourage drooling – an important point.

The conventional interpretation in the literature of these scenes is that the hyenas are being fattened for human consumption. However, the author proposes an alternative theory, namely that hyena saliva is being collected and administered to other animals in an attempt at veterinary medicine.

Keywords: hyena, immunity, animal-diseases, birds, cattle, dogs, vets, medicine-pellets

Teti cemetery scenes of hyenas in captivity during Old Kingdom

Pictorial evidence of the force-feeding of hyenas, first appears in 5th Dynasty reign of Nyuserra (circa 2445 – 2421 BCE) tomb of Ti. Ti's duties included being the administrator of the royal poultry estates. Harpur and Scremin (2006, p. 404) report similar scenes which appear in the 6th Dynasty Teti pyramid complex, in the tombs of Kagemni, Mereruka, Mereri. Another nearby tomb, that of Inumin, on the bottom register of the North wall, shows two hyenas being manhandled. The scenes on the registers above, depict hunting dogs – all ten wearing collars - tearing apart an ibex (Kanawati 2006, plate 13).

Because of its richness of detail and greater familiarity to tomb visitors, I shall focus primarily on the hyenas in the mastaba of Kagemni. These images have been painstakingly copied with detailed commentary by Harpur and Scremin (2006). Several registers depict scenes of typical daily life; they appear in Room IV on what remains of the West wall, divided into right and left sections: see the line-drawings in Harpur and Scremin (2006, pp. 496- 497).

In the middle register of the right wall, scribes are monitoring the apparent force-feeding of two female hyenas, while a male hyena on a lead is watching. The word ***Ndr**t* meaning 'imprisonment' is written three times describing the three hyenas. The other phrase seems to translate: 'a fraction (*Ro*), or (?) dose, of provisions for Amun'. The next lower register depicts geese and ducks in a large free-range enclosure, and men rolling bread into pellets.

The bottom register of the left wall shows men trapping wild fowl in two large hexagonal nets. The middle register shows a man with a large sack on his shoulder; he is pouring grain into the end of one of the three large square cages, containing many ducks and geese in cramped conditions. The remains of the incomplete top register show a man rolling bread into small pellets, which are being fed to three scrawny ducks who do not seem to object to being handled (Harpur and Scremin 2006, p. 407).

In their detailed commentary to the hyena scenes, we are informed that 'hyenas were fattened as a source of meat for human consumption'. Other noteworthy remarks are:

(i) incised lines below the jaws are 'possibly saliva in anticipation of the food prepared for its benefit';
(ii) of one male and two females, it is only the females shown as being force-fed;
(iii) 'fowls were plucked and trimmed for hyenas';
(iv) As a chunk of food approaches the female hyena, 'she seems to be drooling';
(v) 'The impression received by the viewer is that the hyena's saliva-producing glands are functioning at an abnormal rate'.

(Harpur and Scremin 2006, pp. 404- 405).

It is the author's hypothesis that the object of the force-feeding, likely with spoiled meat, was not to fatten an already fat hyena; it was precisely to encourage the excessive salivation of the fasting hyena, for reasons discussed *infra.*

The wall relief originally found in Mereruka's mastaba has comparable and some additional features (see image Germond 2001, plate 29). Two hyenas are each being force-fed some sort of large pellet; there are also descriptive hieroglyphs. Over each hyena appears the caption '**wsA**' meaning 'fat', or 'fatten' (depending on whether **wsA** is taken as an adjective or infinitive verb form) next to the word '***HXt***' identifying 'hyena'. This same simple text is also captioned for the hyena 'force-feeding' scene in Inumin's tomb (Kanawati 2006, plate 13). However, consideration ought to be given for another meaning of the word '**wsA**' which is 'to dry up' (Gardiner: 562). This action on the part of the hyena handler implies another intention altogether – namely by judicious use of a tampon to swab the hyenas' mouth secretions. Notwithstanding, the **wsA** hyenas in both of these two tombs already appear to be fat! And to reiterate, in the tomb of Kagemni (Harpur and Scremin 2006, p. 496) showing force-feeding, the descriptive word before the word hyena is ***Ndrt***, not 'fatten', but 'imprisoned'.

In Mereruka's tomb the food in the hyenas' sight is not nicely trussed; rather it is a disorderly array of dead ducks, meat on the bone, leg meat and ribs, numbering fourteen items in all – seemingly, prestigious offering food that has spoilt. Breasted and Allen writing their guest foreword to the publication of the tomb of Mereruka, poetically describe the animal figures as 'often crowded together in violent motion' (Duell 1938, p. xii). The bird feeding scenes in Mereruka (Duell 1938, plate 52) shows, on the bottom register, twenty-five apparently healthy cranes eagerly feeding on grain from the sack of an attendant. The middle register shows three men feeding pellets to lethargic ducks. The top register seems to show the force-feeding of ducks and geese. Another scene (Duell 1938, plate 53) shows grain being scattered into a large cramped fowl enclosure. In contrast, a contemporaneous code of good practice can be seen in southern Egypt, as segregated cranes and geese in spacious enclosures are scatter-fed grain in the Deir el Gebrawi tomb of 'Aba' (actually *Ibi*) an occupant who happened to know 'all the secret magic' (de G. Davies, 1902, plate XVI).

Egyptologists' views on hyenas

In her Ph.D. thesis on meat production in ancient Egypt, Salima Ikram makes a passing comment about the conventional belief, which she attributes to von Bissing in 1905, that the Egyptians tried to domesticate hyenas for human consumption. This claim is based solely on the strength of the depiction of the hyenas as being tied up in enclosures near farmyards (Ikram 1995, p. 6). She comments that hyenas are never mentioned in food or offering lists, and if eaten, the Egyptians were the only people in the ancient world to have done this. However, in her subsequent publications, as the leading authority in the bioarchaeology of ancient Egypt, Ikram (2001 and 2003) falls in with the general consensus that hyenas were indeed eaten by humans.

Hyenas are described by Osborn and Osbornova (1998, p. 97) as carrion eaters with powerful jaws and teeth, capable of crushing the bones of larger animals. No other animal can extract nutrients from dry bones as can the hyena. It swallows sharp bone fragments, which can rattle in its stomach, then to be excreted as powdery calcium or regurgitated as indigestible pellets (Kingdon 1991, p. 96). In dental morphology, hyenas have massive premolars used to crack bone, in association with their cat-like carnassial tooth used to slice flesh, hair and muscle with ease (van Valkenburgh 1996, p. 242). Chewing bones is injurious to teeth (as sabretooth cats found to their cost) whereas hyenas keep their carnassial tooth (looking very much like Gardiner's hieroglyph N34) sharp by not cracking bone with it (van Valkenburgh 1996, p. 242).

Hyenas are easily kept in captivity and will reproduce there, living 15 – 25 years. Striped hyenas (*Hyaena hyaena*) are the species most shown in ancient Egyptian art. There are also depictions of the Spotted hyena (*Crocuta crocuta*), with their characteristic rounded ears. A later example is to be found in the 18th Dynasty tomb of Antef. For noting the difference between the two types of hyena see Evans (2010: 116-117). The hyenas in question show neither spots nor stripes, however, John Watt (personal communication 23 Sept. 2018) would have identified the hyenas in Kagemni's tomb as spotted hyenas due to their shape and bulk size. Hyenas can become very tame to those who attend the animal from its early months (Legge 2011, p. 616). Legge (2011, p. 615) considers the interpretation offered by Margaret Murray in 1905, to the effect that domesticated hyenas were fed clean and wholesome food so they could be eaten. Curiously, Osborn and Osbornova (1998, Fig.7-157) show a copy image from the 5th Dynasty Giza tomb of Seshahotep, which depicts a labelled offering list line-up of 14 heads, including the head of a hyena, together with waterfowl, cattle, oryx, gazelle. In another 5th Dynasty tomb, the chapel of Sekhem-ankh-ptah at Saqqara, there is another depiction of an obviously tamed young hyena being carried by an offering bearer, next to another offering bearer carrying, according to the hieroglyph label, a white-fronted goose. This goose was sacred to the god Geb and often thought to be the primordial 'Great Cackler' (Legge 2011, p. 616).

But the question remains open for Legge as to the claimed custom of hyena meat being used for human food, whether killed in a hunt, or carefully fattened under husbandry. He points out the wastefulness of feeding animal flesh to a hyena, rather than simply eating the game animal itself. As well, he questions the need to force-feed a hyena, given their notorious habit of gorging to satiety whenever suitable food is available; the hyena can eat 1/3 of its own body weight in one feeding (Legge 2011, p. 616).

Hyenas in Kenya

Hyenas are descended from carrion-feeding ancestors and today are Africa's most successful predator. The Maasai word for hyena means 'to eat greedily' or 'the gluttonous one' (Flies 2017). Andrew Flies has carried out immunological research into why hyenas do not exhibit several types of disease-induced mortality that are common in other animals (Flies 2012, pp. 110-119). He collaborates with Kay Holekamp (2009, pp. 461-471) who has for 25 years studied hyenas in Kenya. A summary of their research, published in 'The Conservation' (19 April 2017) that may hold relevance to one of ancient Egypt's species of hyena - the Spotted or 'laughing hyena' (*Crocuta crocuta*) is as follows:

(I) Although exposed to many pathogens, hyenas appear to be unaffected by the bacteria of putrefaction and disease;
(II) They are unlikely to carry rabies or canine distemper, viruses which kill lions, wild dogs, foxes and other carnivores;
(III) The immune system of wild hyenas is more robust than that of those in captivity, and is stronger in females than in males;
(IV) The cleanliness (or not) of their surroundings bears strongly on the effectiveness of their immune defences.

Rabies in Ptahhotep's desert world?

As previously noted, two hyenas being 'force fed' in the tomb of Inumin, are on the wall predominantly showing the activities of hunting dogs. On the North wall (see Kanawati 2006, plate 25) a seated Inumin has his hunting dog under the chair together with a tied-up pet monkey who clambers all over the docile dog. On the West wall, a similar situation of below-chair activity shows that a *painting* of a naked child has been placed next to the incised relief of the hunting dog (Kanawati 2006, p. 40).

In a general comment about Egyptian dogs as pets, Janssen and Janssen (1989, p. 11) report that dogs are never shown being fondled or played with by children, perhaps because of a fear of bites, and canine rabies. Striking terror for more than 4,000 years, rabies has been described as the world's most diabolical virus (Wasik and Murphy 2012). Any ancient Egyptian was susceptible – all it took was a bite from the Pharaoh's infected hunting dog, or from getting too close to the carriers of rural rabies such as the jackal, fox, mongoose or genet.

Such a scenario - of life-threatening dangers lurking in Seth's realm – takes on more intense meaning when we reconsidered a familiar scene from the tomb of Ptahhotep. The East Wall panorama scene of Ptahhotep's chapel has seven registers of seasonal activities. The double register of the wall's middle register features a 'Desert hunt' scene with an assembly of prey, predators, and pests (the locust), and carnivores mating amidst the *materia medica* vegetation of the savannah plants. Included in the scene is Khnumhotep walking ahead of hyenas and dogs on leads. On a sub upper register, the two hyenas are led by rope, while their untethered cub follows; in the underneath register, the four hunting dogs are led by leads attached to their choke-collars (Harpur and Scremin 2008, p. 172, Fig. 241). On the left-hand upper sub-register, one of the hunting dogs bites the ear of one of two hyenas next to him. This hyena turns back its head and licks at the neck of the aggressive dog (see Harpur and Scremin 2008, p. 113, Fig. 161). At the opposite end of this register, oblivious to savage dogs let loose, is a pair of mating foxes, described by Harpur and Scremin (2008, p. 108, Fig.151) as 'dribbles of foam' coming from the jaws of the copulating foxes. Rabies indeed!

Veterinary medicine

Bearing in mind that depiction of human illness in ancient Egypt is rare, the depiction of sick animals is almost completely lacking (Lord 2010, p. 94). The only known papyrus, sadly incomplete, that has been found relating to the medical treatment of animals is the Kahun Veterinary Papyrus (Petrie Museum UC32036) found during Petrie's excavation of the Middle Kingdom town at Lahun. The surviving fragments deal with three case studies of ailing bulls. The difficulty of identifying the diseases arises from the generality of the described symptoms, and the challenges of the language.

Concentrations of livestock would have rendered the herds liable to recurring plagues of environmental origin, e.g. anthrax (Lord 2010: 96). Thus, animal diseases that affected the food supply would have been a serious problem for ancient Egyptian society. Also, animal diseases have negative impacts on human health, when they are capable of transmission to humans (Lord 2010: 97). Lord also reminds us that many wild animals contain zoonotic diseases (illnesses that can be transferred to humans).

It is interesting to seek an explanation from the array of agricultural animals in the 5th Dynasty Giza tomb of Nefer (Figure 1 after *Illustration 14* Junker: 1943, p.59). The top register shows cranes and geese. The middle register labels four different 'oxen'. The bottom register shows four handlers with tamed wild animals. The oryx and ibex handlers appear to be putting something in the mouths of their charges. The hyena minder appears to be patting the back of his charge, or possibly he is after the hyena's unique anal gland secretion. It is to be noted that all the birds and animals can predispose to various contagions, except the guardian hyena.

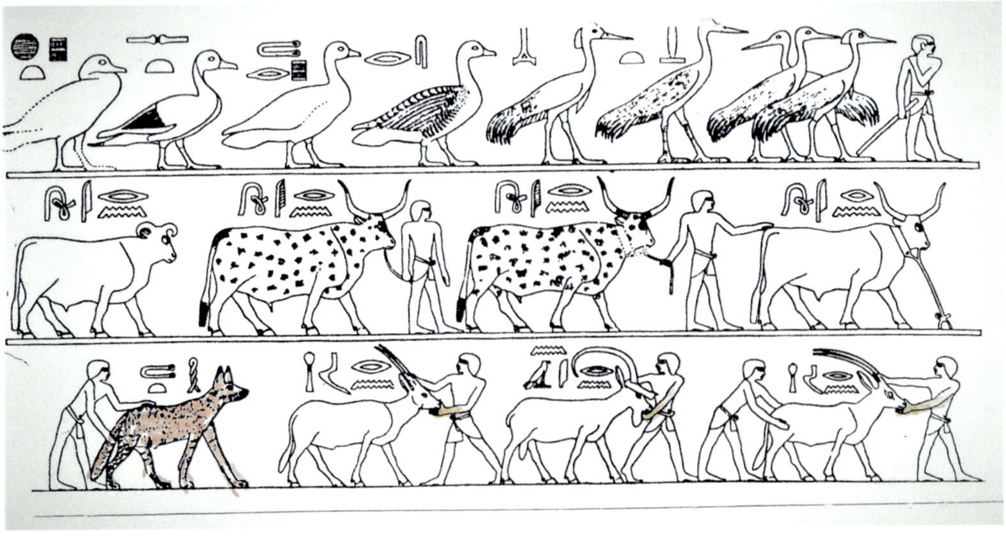

Figure 1. 5th Dynasty tomb of Nefer. Scene of important birds and animals which predispose to infection, with a tamed hyena known to have disease resistance. After Junker (1943:59).

A suggestion: how treatment was administered to ailing fowl

Modern life knows only too well about poultry diseases, such as salmonella, and the drastic measures that must be taken to combat bird flu outbreaks. When wild birds are crowded and stressed due to habitat loss or other factors, outbreaks of coccidiosis and other parasitic conditions are known to increase. Generally, birds kept in captivity can develop either of two strains of the high mortality coccidiosis, intestinal or renal; both lead to reduced egg production, weight loss and death unless early treatment with medicated feed (sulphonamides) and care to keep their surroundings hygienic (Atkinson *et al* 2009, p. 173). Wild water-fowl, especially ducks, geese and cormorants, all depicted in the ancient Egyptian art work, would surely have been prone to earlier viral strains of renal coccidian infection, while captive cranes and other water-fowl may have succumbed to avian tuberculosis – a bacterial infection – as they still do now. In the hot summer of 2018, drought affected many UK wetlands, and there were news reports of large numbers of geese falling ill with botulism from the toxic algae on dried up ponds.

Even with no knowledge of modern science, the Egyptians could still recognise that groups of humans, as well as birds, lions or dogs, could all mysteriously die; the rationale was put down to 'malevolent spirits and various demons taking possession of a body' (Walker 1996, p. 108). When a large outbreak of an illness occurred, and threatened to overwhelm the population, it seems likely that diseased or dead carcasses, whether human or animal, were not always disposed of hygienically. Scavenging hyenas may well have moved in to clean up. In desert ecosystems where decomposition is inhibited by aridity, the hyena – known to dig up buried bodies – plays a unique part in using, breaking down and recycling rare and precious organic matter (Kingdon 1991, p. 96). At some point, curiosity would have been aroused by the seeming survival strength and immunity of the laughing demonic scavenger creature. Early medical theorists experimented with the concept of 'treating like to cure like'; it seems fair to assume that pioneers of veterinary practice would have thought likewise. The Egyptians revered goose gods, in particular, the cosmic laughing 'Great Cackler', the description which best fits the White-fronted goose (*Anser albifrons*) – known, as said before, to be the avatar of the god Geb – which is much featured in the water-fowl scenes of Kagemni. Is it not at least plausible that reasoned like-to-cure-like methodology would have led the ancients to attempt to stop illness in fowl by resort to the powers of the hyena?

Oral administration of cures was already known; contemporaneous Pyramid Texts tell of the ritual cleansing of the mouth with natron pellets. And much is made of the notion that gulping down the magic of powerful beings will transfer their magic and power to the King's belly (Utterances, 273-4; Faulkner's translation). In a 5th Dynasty scene (Berlin 14642) showing the force feeding of cranes and geese in the tomb of Sopdu-hotep, some enlightening text is provided. Two migratory geese plus a resident goose are named, and the poultry handler seems to be saying (Figure 2): (hieroglyphs ***bd***) this 'natron' (bread-pellet) is a ***weapon*** (hieroglyph N34) to treat your exhausted/weakened condition (presumably after the long migratory flight these birds make). The man administering the pellet uses a physician's pot. The earliest designation of doctor is simply an arrow, as in the 3rd Dynasty wooden panel of Hesi-ra (Nunn 1996, p. 115). The sign of 'two arrows shown in a quiver' on two Middle Kingdom coffins indicate their status as doctors (Nunn 1996, p. 115). Similarly, in the Old Kingdom wall scenes, the occupation of 'scribe' would be implied by pictographs of reed brush, bowl for water, and a rectangular palette with two ink cakes.

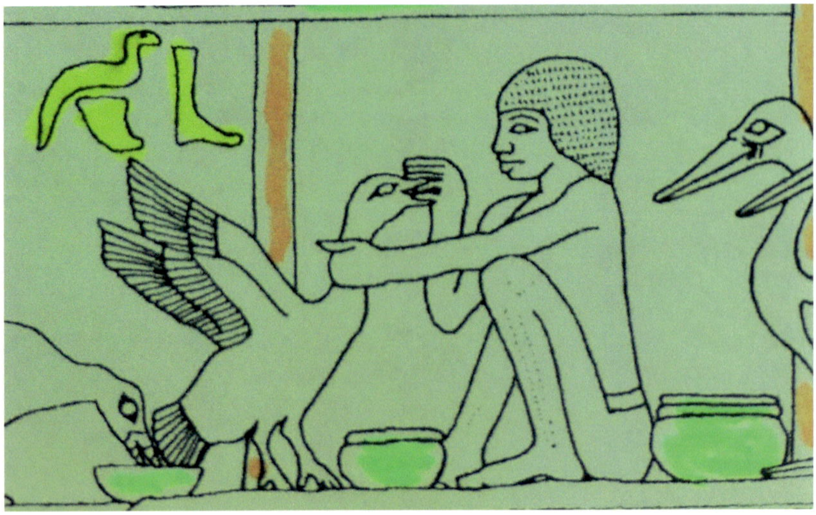

Figure 2. 5th Dynasty tomb of Sopduhotep. Speech bubble claims to give a 'weapon'-treatment (N34: a hyena tooth, rather than bronze ingot) for the exhaustion of the migratory ***trp*** goose. After Wreszinski (1923-1938) *Atlas III*, Pl. 83.

Perhaps more should be read into the art-work on the bow case of Tutankhamun, with a correlation to the troubled times of disease morbidity during the Amarna Period - what Kemp (2012, p. 228) repeatedly calls 'pestilence' whilst Kozloff (2006, pp. 26-46) argues more strongly for Kemp's pestilence to be plague. In four vignettes (see Burton photographs in the Griffith Institute) animals - amidst savannah plants (including an ibex eating henbane) – hyenas, antelopes, hares are brought down with arrows; however (on the left-hand Obverse scene), one female hyena holds an arrow in her mouth. Recovered from the Aten Temple is a *talatat*-block showing a fleeing desert hunt victim which happens to be a female hyena being chased (see *National Geographic* Nov. 1970: 650 - 651). In the 18th Dynasty tomb of Rekhmire, a wounded hyena pulls at a bent arrow in its bleeding chest. Osborn and Osbornova (1998, p. 100) state that, throughout the Pharaonic period, the hyena ***clawing*** an arrow in either its mouth, neck or chest, was a popular theme. Right back to the 5th Dynasty and a scene from the funerary temple of Sahure, the hyena uses its paws to remove from its mouth the huntsman's arrow (see Ikram 2001, Figure 4, p.131).

Just as the symbolism of the arrow, plus pot, designated the tools and title of the Egyptian doctor (*swnw*); I would like to suggest that the 'claw-like' or 'hyena carnassial tooth shape' hieroglyph **N34** - known to be a copper or bronze weapon - together with the ***Nw*** pot were the emblem 'tools of trade' used to denote the occupation of veterinary doctor during the Old Kingdom. Gardiner's N34 weapon-hieroglyph is surely the best antiquarian root to be found for later generations of doctors choosing war-themed dialogue in reference to disease and treatment.

'Better far an open, whose attacks can be met, than a hidden foe, who, invisible, deals his death blows with an unsparing hand, and creates a wail through the length and breadth of the (Egyptian) land' (Hunter 1883, p. 49). These words were written by the Surgeon-General, Sir Guyer Hunter following his investigation of the outbreak of plague in June 1883 at the Damietta branch of the Nile. His report to Her Majesty's Government revealed that this cholera, not from

India as rumoured, but arose locally as cholera was already endemic in Egypt from at least 1865. Hunter's epidemiology research found that the documented previous outbreaks of Egyptian cholera followed herds of cattle wiped out by typhus epidemics. One of his curious findings stated that the local population knew a cholera epidemic was imminent, as sparrows deserted the towns, and did not return until the epidemic was in decline (Hunter 1883, p. 61). Which brings me back to the ancestor Egyptians critically observant of their natural environment especially when it came to working out attributes connecting bird symbols to the language. Interestingly, according to Gardiner (1988 p. 471), the sparrow hieroglyph (G37) is used as the determinative for the words 'ill' and 'diseased'.

The two men administering the geese and cranes in Sopdu-hotep's tomb were a class above the average 'poultry handlers', and in the likely service of the king (note splendid columns for a non-typical bird aviary in the background). In any case, as well as the logic of building up the lost muscle weight of birds after epic flight journeys, the Old Kingdom poultry experts may also have stumbled upon the idea of using an animal weapon potion – what we would call 'vaccine' - as disease prevention or cure. Not the actual hyena's *claw* tooth, but the source of where the status tooth grew and the copious **saliva** which could be harvested to treat outbreaks of incoming avian disease. A serious and uncontained outbreak could have led to economic collapse, and in some quarters, likely food privation or starvation. This would hardly have been a propitious time for people to give their limited supply of fowl to gluttonous hyenas held captive in the farm enclosure.

Carob cure adjunct suggestion

The hieroglyphic word for carob is Nedjem *ndm* (Germer 2008, p. 151). The carob tree tree (*Ceratonia siliqua*) can grow to 50 feet and, if not cut down by the *medjeh* wood-workers for its high quality hardwood, would continue to bear fruit for 80-100 years. Usage of carob wood for planks in boat building is attested on the eastern wall of the offering room in Ti's tomb.

From an examination of the hundreds of prescriptions in the ancient Egyptian medical papyri, it is clear that many of the internal medicines prescribed for humans were medicated foods, such as bread, cakes, or sweet beer (Walker 1996, p. 109). Rather than using emmer or barley, flour for the treatment bread more than likely came from the carob bean – an animal-fodder crop, also known today to be an effective remedy to treat intestinal disease in human infants. The drug-like compound of carob fruit (90% pulp, 10% seed producing a bean gum, high in sugar and condensed tannins) is today widely used for pharmaceutical purposes as it is linked with the inhibition of gastrointestinal diseases, and a good carrier agent (Goulas 2016).

In a register of the Room 4, North wall of Kagemni (Harpur and Scremin 2006, p. 182) subjects are shown bringing goods to trade for carob oil or carob beer out of distinctive shaped containers (the tall oil vessel known as Gardiner's hieroglyph W1) and the smaller ***m3t*** granite pot with handles (Gardiner's hieroglyph W7). The caption says: ***ndt Ht*** (almost the word for hyena!) with the determinative of carob beans. Harpur and Scremin (2006, p. 429) provide us with their happy translation of: 'The craftsmen have received a great amount of sweet oil'. I think the translation needs to be more literal and realistic along the lines of: 'the poor serfs (***ndt***) are bringing along their worldly goods in exchange for carob rations (as the emmer and barley wheat are no longer available)'.

My suggestion would be that inferior carob bread ought to have been the obvious medium with which to soak up the salivation of a fasting hyena with induced drooling at the sight of nearby poultry carcasses. Thence this medicated bread, infused with whatever magical disease-fighting powers the hyena possessed to make him only liable to die from the arrow or old age, was given to birds to enhance their survival. Either as a curative or a preventative and whether efficacious or not, we cannot know for certain.

Famine as a driver of desperate measures?

The images featuring the role of the desert survivor hyena in captivity that I have examined are all from between the 5th and 6th Dynasties. The 5th Dynasty came to an end in the reign of Unas. Famines naturally occur as the result of low Nile risings over several years, and the breakdown of orderly administration would also contribute. In passing, I would mention from the famous causeway of Unas, the haunting scenes of naked starving Bedouins. Seemingly these pictures, which were not hidden in a sealed tomb nor displayed on a temple wall, were left as a monument for public scrutiny as some sort of commemoration or future warning. Typically, Bedouin are the people most adept at surviving the harshest desert environments. However, some Old Kingdom natural and/or man-made disasters (that no one's really sure of) contributed towards savannah becoming hostile desert. Did indiscriminate over-hunting by Pharaoh's men with rabid dogs put a nail in the carob wood coffin by destroying the delicate landscape?

Desperate times, as when disease causes the poultry and cattle food chain to break down, needed desperate remedies. Extraction of magical hyena saliva for bird medication purposes, and other veterinary procedures, began (as far as the chronology allows) in the tomb of Ti, who had amongst his many important titles Administrator of the Royal Poultry Estates.

Summary

Early Egyptology scholars interpreted the tomb art showing hyenas forcibly held down with some sort of activity taking place at their drooling mouths as 'force-feeding'. This led to the unchallenged assumption that ancient Egyptians in their desert hunt expeditions captured hyenas in order to rear and eat their meat. Seeing other sympatric carnivores e.g. lions, fox and dogs - all prone from time to time to populations decimation through anthrax, rabies and other viral diseases - has led this author to an alternate theory. This theory was inspired by the outcome of testing hyena antibody responses (as disclosed in recent public media announcements of Flies in *The Conversation* 19 April 2017) that hyenas are known to survive all such outbreaks. Given the fragility of the Egyptian pastoral economy, it is not beyond the realms of imagination that, when the Old Kingdom Egyptians came across flocks of dead birds, dead antelope and cattle herds, they were mocked by healthy hyenas eating everything in sight. Surely the priests and farmers accredited some sort of magical ichor in the make-up of the laughing surviving hyena.

Recapping the method shown in the various tombs discussed, two assistants have the hogtied female hyena in the submissive role on her back while her male partner looks on. The operator keeps one hand on the hyena's throat; the fingers of his other hand delicately dip some bread-pellets to mop up the stated mouth droolings – which today we know contain antibodies resistant to animal infectious diseases. Hyenas eat any kind of good, or bad, food and do not require force-feeding to gorge their insatiable appetite. However, as food supplier workers saw their precious flocks succumb, the Egyptian leaders choose to combat the deadly foe of pestilence by symbolic use of a hyena's tooth – or in actual practice the saliva that the tooth rose out of - as their *weapon* of attack. With the hyena's razor-sharp teeth, this is a very dangerous job for the farm-yard handlers or, in accordance with my surmise – Old Kingdom specialised veterinary doctor practitioners. As the modern medical saying goes, the riskiest vaccine is the one not given.

Bibliography

Atkinson, C, Thomas, N and Hutes, B 2009. *Parasitic Diseases of Wild Birds.* Wiley, London.

de G. Davies, N 1902. *The Rock Tombs of Deir el Gebrawi.* Egypt Exploration Fund, London.

Evans, L 2010. *Animal Behaviour in Egyptian Art.* A.C.E. Studies 9, Aries and Phillips, London.

Flies, A 2017. 'Spotted hyenas rarely die from disease: we set out to discover why' in *The Conversation* online, 19 April 2017.

Flies, A *et al* 2012. *Development of a hyena immunology toolbox* in *Veterinary Immunology* 2012, #145, 110-119.

Gardiner, A 1988. *Egyptian Grammar.* Griffith Institute, Oxford.

Germer, R 2002. *Die Heilpflanten der Agypter.* Artemis and Winkler, Dusseldorf.

Goulas, V 2016. *Functional Components of Carob Fruit: Linking the Chemistry and Biological Space* in *International Journal of Molecular Sciences* 2016 Nov, 17 (11).

Harpur, Y and Scremin, P 2008. *The Chapel of Ptahhotep.* Oxford Expedition to Egypt, Oxford.

Harpur, Y and Scremin, P 2006. *The Chapel of Kagemni.* Oxford Expedition to Egypt, Oxford.

Hunter, G 1884. *Remarks on the Epidemic of Cholera in Egypt.* Report to Her Majesty's Government.

Ikram, S 1995. *Choice cuts: meat production in Ancient Egypt.* Cairo.

Ikram, S 2001 *The Iconography of the Hyena in Ancient Egypt* in *MDAIK*, Vol.57, pp.127-140.

Junker, H 1943. *Giza 6: Die Mastabas des Nefer, Kedfi, Kahjef und die westlich anschliessenden Grabanlagen.* Holder-Pichler-Tempsky, Vienna.

Kanawati, N 2006 *The Teti Cemetery at Saqqara Vol. VIII The Tomb of Inumin.* The Australian Centre for Egyptology: Reports 24.

Kemp, B 2012 *The City of Akhenaten and Nefertiti Amarna and its People.* Thames and Hudson, London.

Kingdon, J 1991 *Arabian Mammals: A Natural History.* Academic Press, Bahrain.

Kozloff, A 2006 *Bubonic Plague in the reign of Amenhotep III?* in Kmt 17, #3, 36-46.

Legge, A 2011 *The Hyaena in Dynastic Egypt: Fancy Food or Fantasy Food?* pp.613-621 in *Int. J. Osteoarchaeol.* John Wiley and Sons. Published 5 May 2010 in Wiley Online Library.

Lord, C 2010 *The man who knows bulls: veterinary practice in Ancient Egypt* in ed. J. Cockitt and R. David *Pharmacy and Medicine in Ancient Egypt.* BAR, Oxford.

Nunn, J 1996. *Ancient Egyptian Medicine.* British Museum Press, London.

Van Valkenburgh, B 1996. *Feeding Behaviour in Free Ranging Large African Carnivores* in *Journal of Mammalogy* Vol. 77, #1 (Feb 1996), 240-254.

Walker, J 1996. *Food, Health and Disease in Ancient Egypt* pp.101-114 in ed. Gae Callender *Aegyptiaca Essays on Egyptian Themes.* Macquarie Ancient History Association, Sydney.

Wasik, B and Murphy, M 2012. *Rabid.* Viking.

Watts, H and Holekamp, K 2009. *Ecological Determinants of Survival and Reproductions in the Spotted Hyena* in *Journal of Mammalogy* 2009, #90, 461-471.

Bone Identification and Angulometry of the Foot and Ankle in Egypt's Mummies

Patrícia Rodríguez Corbera
oatroco@gmail.com
Podiatry, University of Barcelona
Berta Torrents Pérez
Podiatry, University of Barcelona
Pablo Martínez-Escauriaza Peral, Rosa Dinarès Solà
Autonomous University of Barcelona
Jesús Herrerín López
Autonomous University of Madrid

Abstract: Introduction: The ancient Egyptian culture specialized in the art of medicine, being able to perfect the techniques of mummification. Mummified bodies reproduce the appearance of the living, but their internal structures are retracted. Podiatry, a science that was born in ancient Egypt, can provide their knowledge to study changes in the structure of the foot and ankle after mummification. **Materials and Methods:** Nine cases of mummified lower extremities (LE) were analyzed. The different bones were identified and the stature of six of the individuals was studied, as well as the age of one of them. Different angles of the foot and ankle were assessed, and a pathological diagnostic study was carried out. **Results:** Of the cases analyzed, 100% of the rearfoot and midfoot bones were present. In 28.57% of the cases, the proximal phalanges were broken and the medial and distal were missing. The mean height of the adults was 164.07cm (SD ± 5.02) for hypothetical men and 161.37cm (SD ± 5.42) for hypothetical women. The majority of altered angles indicated an elevation of the plantar arch (cavus foot). The most observed pathologies were incipient osteoarthritis (85.75%), Haglund's deformity (57.14%) and spur (42.86%). **Discussion and Conclusions:** Fractures of the phalanges are due to spoliation, while the deformation in cavus of the feet can be due to tissue retraction. The superposition and quality of the radiographs affects their study, creating biases in the measurement. A podiatric protocol can improve the study of mummified LE.

Keywords: Forensic podiatry, anthropology, mummification, angulometry.

Introduction

From the remotest times of humanity, facing death, with the consequent complete extinction of the individual, has been a challenge to the nature and philosophy of man, who has always preferred to believe in a definitive survival after death. The ancient Egyptians were not an exception, and they went to eccentric extremes to ensure the physical survival of the posthumous body.

It is believed that the first Egyptians buried their dead naked or wrapped in sheets in shallow graves, where heat and dry air mummified the body (Sluglett, 1990). This fact did not go unnoticed by later generations, nourishing their beliefs and hopes about eternal life after death, consequently giving rise to artificial mummification.

PHARMACY AND MEDICINE IN ANCIENT EGYPT
(ARCHAEOPRESS 2021): 88–103

Thanks to the Egyptians' dedication to preservation over time, nowadays we can document many of the foundations of medical science that were established in Egypt more than five thousand years ago.

The ancient Egyptian society has always had a wide reputation for medical knowledge, documented in several papyruses, as that of Edwin Smith, or interpreted in the different polychrome scenes that surround some tombs, such as those of Ank-ma-hor and Niankhkhnum, in Saqqara (Harpur and Scremin, 2010). It is in these same tombs where the first signs of foot care are observed.

Although literature has rarely highlighted the importance of this practice in the Egyptian culture, scenes found in Saqqara, Abu Seir, El-Bersha, Beni Hassan, El-Hammamiya and Thebes show that feet health was important for this historic society (El-Kilany, 2017), which leads us to think that the origin of podiatry dates back to ancient Egypt.

Podiatry has evolved to become a full medical discipline, specializing in everything related to the foot and ankle. That is why, almost five thousand years later, we return to the place of our beginnings to investigate the techniques of mummification and how they affect the structure of the foot.

Hypothesis and Objectives

The hypothesis raised has been studied with point two of the list of objectives set, and is the following:

'Bandages used in mummification retract the foot and ankle structures.'

The present study is based on the resolution of diverse purposes, all of them from the images given by the 'PROYECTO PANHESI TT16, LUXOR, EGIPTO' (PP-TT16).

1. Identification and description of the bones of the foot and ankle.
2. Value the radiologic angles of the foot and ankle.
3. Detection and diagnosis of pathological signs on foot and ankle bones.
4. Implement a radiological protocol for the study and evaluation of lower extremities (LE) of mummified human samples.

Materials and Methods

The Tomb of Panehsy

The Theban Necropolis lies west of the Egyptian city of Luxor, and that is where the most important mortuary temples of the dynasties XVIII, XIX and XX were built. This necropolis is divided into three zones: The Valley of the Kings, the Valley of the Queens, and the Valley of the Nobles (Betrò *et al.* 2009).

The Valley of the Nobles is formed by six necropolises in which there are buried high officials, nobles, members of the royal family and priests. To the northeast of the temple of Hatshepsut is located Dra Abu al-Naga (FIGURE 1), a necropolis with 17 tombs of pharaohs and 114 of high ranking officials (Porter and Moss, 2004). One of the most outstanding tombs of this region

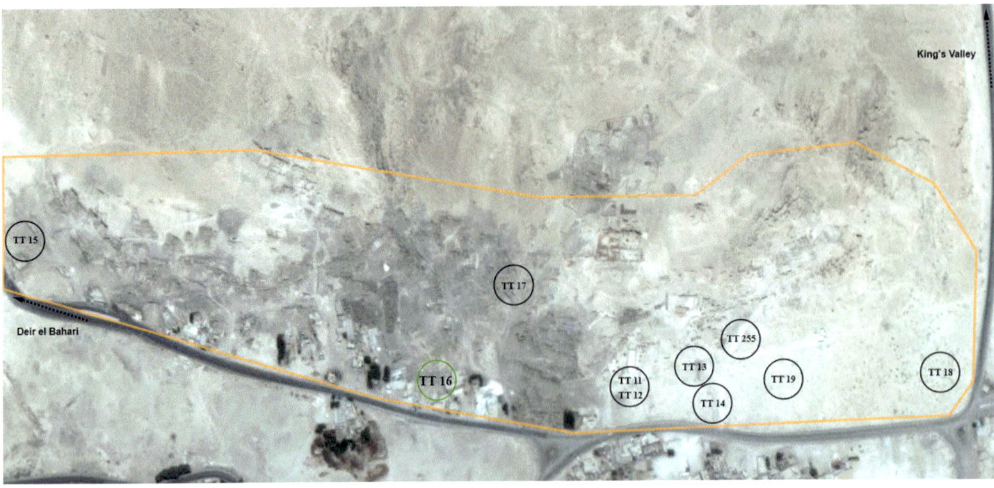

Figure 1: Location of Thebas Tombs in Dra Abu al-Naga. Own elaboration picture.

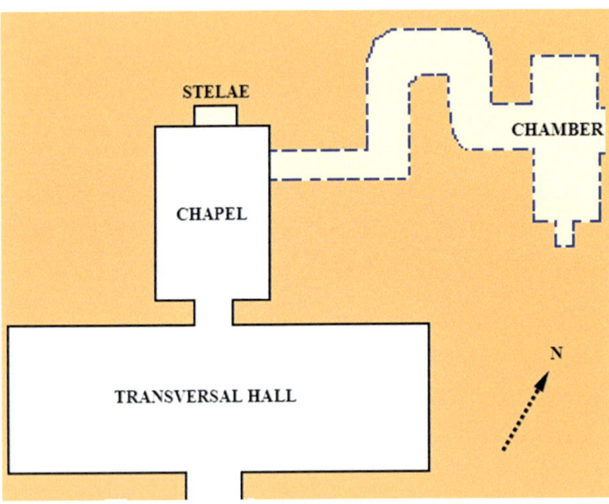

Figure 2: Schematic plan of the Panehsy Tomb. Own elaboration picture.

is the Tomb of Thebes 16 (TT 16), where Panehsy ([hieroglyphs]) was buried. He was a prophet of the court of Amenhotep I, during the second half of the government of Ramesses II, 3rd King of the XIX Dynasty (AD 1293 - 1185) (Porter and Moss, 2004). The tomb is small, about 6.5 m long and 2.3 m deep. It is carved into the rock and consists of two decorated rooms in an inverted T shape, and a passage of 50 m to the funerary pit (FIGURE 2). The paintings on the walls were applied on white plaster and show six painting scenes poorly conserved.

Abundant human remains were found in the path to the burial chamber, among a conglomerate of dust, bandages and pottery, of half a meter in height (FIGURES 3 and 4). This amount of bones is the result of the reuse of the tomb for intrusive burials for more than 1000 years, as well as the continuous plundering by thieves. Although the tomb was built in the XVIII dynasty, it is believed that the remains from the passage are later, from the XXI dynasty (AD 1069 - 945) and forward, to the Third Intermediate Period (Salter-Pedersen, 2004).

The Cases

Among the human remains, some isolated legs were separated for their study. Nine of these samples are included in this study. Technicians photographed them and took x-Ray imaging. The x-Ray equipment used was the ClaroX DR Equino 810 digital direct radiography system,

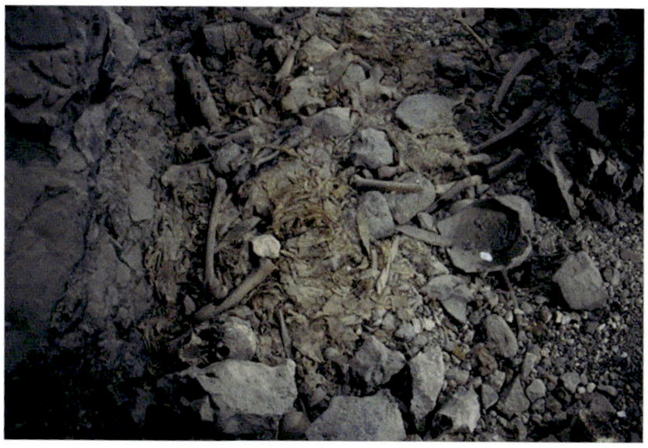

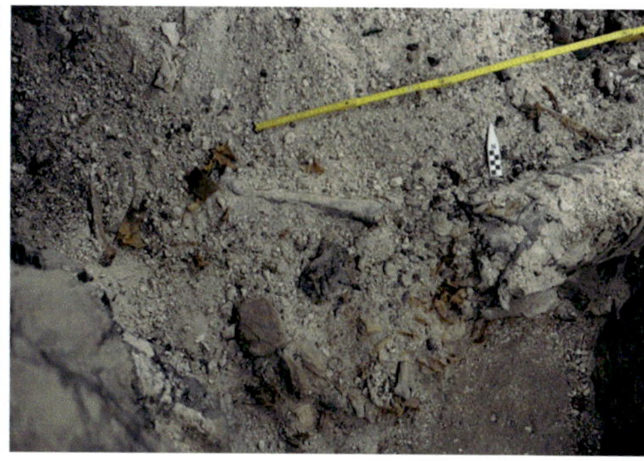

Figures 3 and 4: Bones, dust and pottery in the path of the Panehsy Tomb. Pictures courtesy of PP-TT16.

which consists of a panel connected to a x-ray equipment and to a computer. Its dimensions are 8'x10' and its thickness 15 mm. The characteristics of antero-posterior and dorso-plantar x-ray were 60 Kw and 0.32 mAs, and lateral x-ray were 65 Kv and 0.50 mAs.

Case 1

Case 1 is a sample with human lower extremity appearance. It was found on February 3, 2011 at locus 11/2 of the TT 16, Luxor. It is a right leg and foot with a subchondral cut or break. The calf and the foot were wrapped with linen, as were the toes, which were not separated from each other, but wrapped together. The radiologic studies of this case include two internal oblique projections and two lateral projections of the ankle joint.

Case 2

Case 2 is a sample with human lower extremity appearance. It was found on February 24, 2011 at locus 11/4 of the TT 16, Luxor. It is a right leg and foot with a subchondral cut or break of an adult human. The calf and the foot were wrapped with linen, the toes were wrapped separately. The radiologic studies of this case include one antero-posterior projection and two lateral projections of the ankle joint.

Case 3

Case 3 is a sample with human foot appearance. It was found on February 14, 2011 at locus 11/3.4 of the TT 16, Luxor. It is a right foot, broken above the ankle joint, of an adult human. The foot was wrapped with linen and toes are absent. The radiologic studies of this case include one antero-posterior projection and one lateral projection of the foot.

Case 4

Case 4 is a sample with human lower extremities appearance. It was found on February 14, 2011 at locus 11/4 of the TT 16, Luxor. They are two legs and feet of a subadult human. The left leg has a subchondral cut or break, while the right one retains the entire diaphysis of the femur, along the calf and foot. All toes of both feet are broken. Each leg was wrapped with linen, separately in an initial stage, and together in a later stage. The hallux were wrapped separately, unlike the other toes. The radiologic studies of this case include one antero-posterior projection and one lateral projection of the ankle joints.

Case 5

Case 5 is a sample with human lower extremity appearance. It was found on February 27, 2011 at locus 11/4 of the TT 16, Luxor. It is a right leg and foot, with a subchondral cut or break, of an adult human. The calf and the foot were wrapped with linen, same as the toes, which were wrapped together but broken at the level of phalanges. The bandage was damaged, leaving the mummified skin uncovered. The radiologic studies of this case include one antero-posterior projection of the tibia and fibula and two lateral projections of the ankle joint.

Case 6

Case 6 is a sample with human lower extremity appearance. It was found on February 27, 2011 at locus 11/4 of the TT 16, Luxor. It is a left leg and foot with a subchondral cut or break of an adult human. The calf and the foot were wrapped with linen, same as the toes, which were wrapped together but broken at the level of phalanges. The radiologic studies of this case include one antero-posterior projection of the tibia and fibula, one antero-posterior projection of the ankle joint and two lateral projections of the ankle joint.

Case 7

Case 7 is a sample with human lower extremities appearance. It was found on January third, 2011 at locus 13/1 of the TT 16, Luxor. They are two legs and feet of an adult human, very damaged. The left leg is broken in the distal third of the calf, while the right one retains the entire diaphysis of the tibia and fibula, with a subchondral cut or break. All toes of both feet are broken. Each leg was wrapped with linen, separately in an initial stage, and together in a later stage. The bandage is plentiful and is filled with dirt. The radiologic studies of this case include two antero-posterior projection of the ankle joint, two internal oblique projections of the foot and three lateral projections of the ankle joint.

Case 8

Case 8 is a sample with human lower extremity appearance. It was found on February 23, 2011 at locus 11/4 of the TT 16, Luxor. It is a left leg and foot with a subchondral cut or break of an adult human. The calf and the foot were wrapped with linen. The radiologic studies of this case include one lateral projection of the ankle joint.

Case 9

Case 9 is a sample with human lower extremity appearance. It was found on February 27, 2011 at locus 11/4 of the TT 16, Luxor. It is a right leg and foot of an adult human with a subchondral cut or break. The calf and the foot were wrapped with linen, the toes were wrapped together and the third, fourth and fifth were broken. The radiologic studies of this case include one antero-posterior projection of the tibia and fibula, one intern oblique projection of the foot, and two lateral projections of the ankle joint.

Analysis Methods

Bone Identification

All radiographies have been studied independently, locating and isolating the different bones present in them. Two different methods have been used for this study, both carried out with the design programmes *Gimp 2.0* and *Corel Painter 5.0*. The first method is based on the simple location of each bone, identifying it with a previously assigned letter (FIGURE 5). In the second method, the periphery of the bones was traced, filling the resulting area with an assigned colour (FIGURE 6).

Due to overlapping, cases four and seven were excluded from the bone identification study. An age approximation was calculated in case 4 for being a subadult human, using the skeletal maturity indicators of the foot and ankle described by Hoerr, Pyle, and Francis in 1962. Foot length was also measured, and height approximation was calculated in all cases except in those

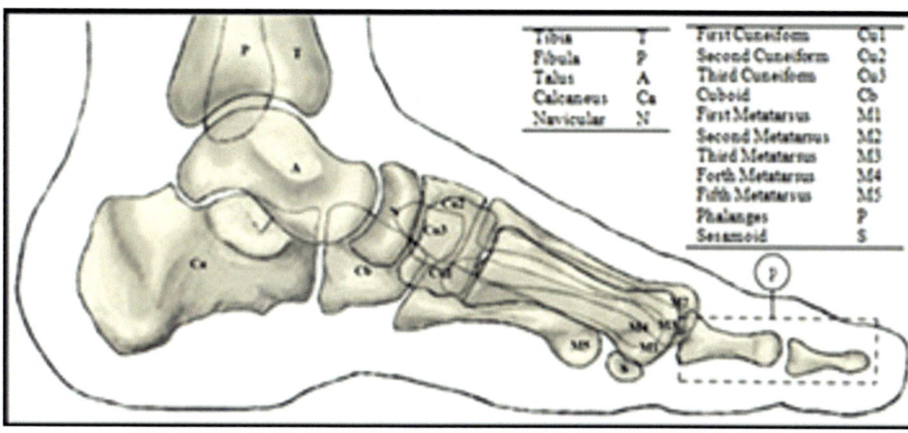

Figure 5: Method of simple bone location. Drawing example. Own elaboration picture.

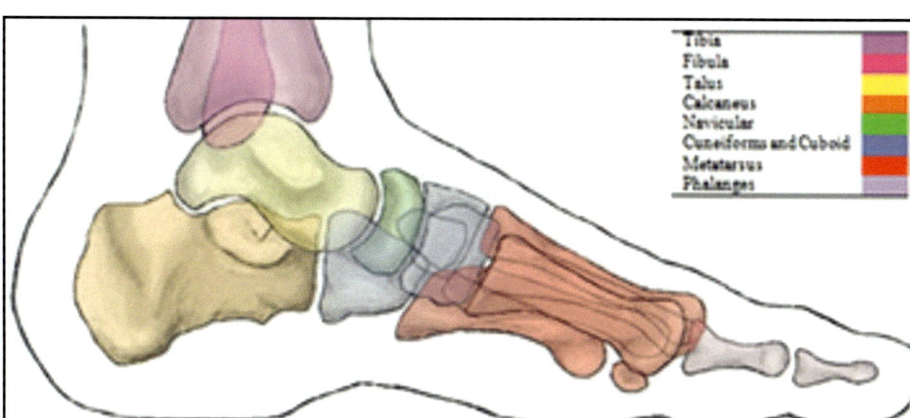

Figure 6: Method of bone area location. Drawing example. Own elaboration picture.

in which tibia was missing. The stature estimation was calculated with the Ratxer *et al.* equation for ancient Egyptians (Raxter *et al.*, 2008). (TABLE 1).

Table 1: Ratxer et al equations

	Equation	SE
Males	2.554*(TL)+69.21	±3.002
Females	2.699*(TL)+61.08	±1.921
Add 2.5 to calculate cadaveric stature[12] **Abbreviations:** TL (Tibial Length); SE (Standard Error).		

Angulometry

To see how the bandages affected the structure of the foot and ankle, a lateral projection x-ray of each case was chosen, on which a total of 16 angles and distances were studied (TABLE 2). All angles were measured with the mathematical software of dynamic geometry *GeoGebra*. Accurate measurements depend on the quality of the radiograph and the accuracy of drawing the angles and reference points described in the consulted bibliography (Berquist, 2017; Christman, 2014; Montage et al., 1984). Due to superposition in cases four and seven, angulometry study was not performed.

Table 2: Angle and given name

1st metatarsal declination angle	1MDA
2nd metatarsal declination angle	2MDA
5th metatarsal declination angle	5MDA
Böhler's angle	BA
Calcaneal inclination angle	CIA
Feiss line	FL
Critical Angle of Gissane	CAG
Hibb's angle	HA
Meary's angle	MA
Internal Moreau-Costa-Bertani's angle	I-MCB
External Moreau-Costa-Bertani's angle	E-MCB
Navicular height	NH
Plantigrade angle	PA
Talar declination angle	TDA
Talo-calcaneal angle	TCA
Tibio-talar angle	TTA

Measurement data were generated and descriptive statistics were calculated for each angle using the statistical software SPSS software package (IBM SPSS Statics for Windows, version 24.0). To assess for significant differences between collected data and normal values, a one-way analysis of variance was conducted with the significance level at $p < 0.05$.

Diagnosis of pathologies

Each radiograph was thoroughly studied for the diagnosis of possible bone diseases, soft tissue pathologies and normal variants. All artefacts seen on radiographs that could have been misleading as pathologies were considered. Percentages were made for pathology found, considering the cases as a population sample of the TT16 tomb. Due to superposition, cases four and seven were not included for diagnosis.

Results

A total of 24 radiographies were analyzed, 21 of these were useful for bone identification. TABLE 3 shows the presence or absence of each bone of the foot and ankle for every case studied. 71.43% were right feet, and 28.57% were left feet. In 100% of cases, talus, navicular, cuboid, calcaneus, cuneiforms and metatarsals were present. Due to overlapping, phalanges weren't evaluable in most cases, being mostly present, but precisely unknown. Tibia and fibula were broken in 14.28% of cases, and proximal phalanges in 28.57%, that is the 100% of evaluable phalanges. Sesamoids were always present, and non accessory bones were identified.

A total of 27 measurements were made in all cases, excluding case 7 due to lack of photomacrographic scale (TABLE 4). 100% of evaluated feet had an Index Minus metatarsal formula, according to a larger 2nd metatarsus.

Foot length mean was 21.60 cm (SD±2.27), being excluded the cases with absence of medial and distal phalanges. Tibial length mean was 36.23 cm (SD±2.01) in adult individuals. An approximation of height was calculated, differentiating the hypothetical sex of the individuals. Hypothetical adult man would measure an average of 164.07 cm (SD±5.02), and hypothetical adult women would measure a mean of 161.37 cm (SD±5.42). For case 4, age approximation was eight to 12 years for a hypothetical man and six to nine for a hypothetical woman, according to tibial, talar and calcaneal morphology.

For the angulometry study, descriptive statics and one-way analysis were calculated (TABLE 5) from a total of 49 angles drawn from seven lateral radiographs, one for each case studied, whose value is collected in TABLE 6. All pathologies and normal variants observed are shown in TABLE 7.

Discussion

Radiographic examination of mummified tissues was applied for the first time by König in 1896. Roentgenology has many advantages, including wide availability, easy access, low cost and high spatial resolution (Panzer *et al.*, 2013). These qualities make it the technique of choice in the field, ahead of laboratory analysis and other imaging studies, such as computed tomography, due to the legal limitation in the handling of the pieces for their transport.

As this is a non-invasive approach to scientific research of mummies, numerous radiographic studies have been made since then to see the behaviour of different tissues during mummification (Rühli *et al.*, 2004; Rühli, 1998; Lynnerup, 2007). The present one being the first to study the changes in the bone configuration of the foot and ankle. The use of bandages and natron, a naturally occurring compound of NaCl, Na_2CO_3, $NaHCO_3$ and NaP_2SO_4 (Smith and Dawson, 2002; Pahl and Parsche, 1991) in the practice of mummification in Ancient Egypt are known from

Table 3: Bone Identification results

			Case1	Case2	Case3	Case5	Case6	Case8	Case9
	Foot		R	R	R	R	L	L	R
	Tibia		+	+	±	+	+	+	+
	Fibula		+	+	±	+	+	+	+
	Talus		+	+	+	+	+	+	+
	Navicular		+	+	+	+	+	+	+
	Cuboid		+	+	+	+	+	+	+
	Calcaneus		+	+	+	+	+	+	+
Cuneiforms	First		+	+	+	+	+	+	+
	Second		+	+	+	+	+	+	+
	Third		+	+	+	+	+	+	+
Metatarsals	First		+	+	+	+	+	+	+
	Second		+	+	+	+	+	+	+
	Third		+	+	+	+	+	+	+
	Forth		+	+	+	+	+	+	+
	Fifth		+	+	+	+	+	+	+
Phalanges	First Ray	Proximal	NE*	NE*	±	NE*	±	NE*	NE*
		Medial	NE*	NE*	–	NE*	–	NE*	NE*
		Distal	NE*	NE*	–	NE*	–	NE*	NE*
	Second Ray	Proximal	NE*	NE*	±	NE*	±	NE*	NE*
		Medial	NE*	NE*	–	NE*	–	NE*	NE*
		Distal	NE*	NE*	–	NE*	–	NE*	NE*
	Third Ray	Proximal	NE*	NE*	±	NE*	±	NE*	NE*
		Medial	NE*	NE*	–	NE*	–	NE*	NE*
		Distal	NE*	NE*	–	NE*	–	NE*	NE*
	Forth Ray	Proximal	NE*	NE*	±	NE*	±	NE*	NE*
		Medial	NE*	NE*	–	NE*	–	NE*	NE*
		Distal	NE*	NE*	–	NE*	–	NE*	NE*
	Fifth Ray	Proximal	NE*	NE*	±	NE*	±	NE*	NE*
		Medial	NE*	NE*	–	NE*	–	NE*	NE*
		Distal	NE*	NE*	–	NE*	–	NE*	NE*
	*In a generic view, most phalanges were present								
Sesamoids	Tibial		+	NE	+	+	+	+	+
	Fibular		+	NE	+	+	+	+	+

Abbreviations: R (Right); L (Left); + (Present); – (Absent); ± (Broken); NE (Not Evaluable).

Table 4: Morphology and lengths studied

						Aprox. Height	
Case	**1st Mtt**	**2nd Mtt**	**Mtt Formula**	**Foot Lenght**	**Tibial Lenght**	**M**	**F**
Case 1	5.49	6.87	Index Minus	20.38	36.42	164.73	161.88
Case 2	5.23	6.72	Index Minus	20.67	32.85	155.61	152.24
Case 3	6.24	6.50	Index Minus	19.28±	NE	NE	NE
Case 4	NE	NE	NE	NE	22.14	128.25	123.33
Case 5	5.19	5.87	Index Minus	20.80	36.50	164.93	162.10
Case 6	6.14	6.71	Index Minus	19.00±	38.08	168.97	166.36
Case 8	5.36	6.41	Index Minus	20.51	NE	NE	NE
Case 9	6.59	7.99	Index Minus	25.65	37.31	NE	NE

Abbreviations: Mtt (Metatarsus); M (Male); F (Female).

Table 5: Statistical results

Angle	Mean	SD	Min-Max	Sig.
1MDA	31.08	5.29	21.07 – 37.25	0.007
2MDA	26.25	3.82	19.22 – 30.78	0.418
5MDA	12.91	4.41	6.78 – 20.20	0.258
BA	28.31	7.08	20.11 – 36.67	0.077
CIA	23.97	2.53	20.15 – 26.27	0.011
FL	19.87	6.07	9.60 – 27.24	0.000
CAG	108.19	5.99	98.92 – 116.36	0.000
HA	139.16	7.56	130.31 – 154.70	0.019
MA	23.00	6.77	9.75 – 31.55	0.001
I-MCB	115.20	8.49	105.69 – 130.49	0.951
E-MCB	139.12	5.10	130.47 – 147.81	0.023
NH	3.74	0.46	3.14 – 4.36	0.006
PA	94.15	7.68	82.16 – 107.43	0.791
TDA	8.77	4.22	2.02 – 14.03	0.000
TCA	32.26	2.94	27.87 – 36.32	0.003
TTA	78.91	9.29	66.45 – 91.13	0.025

Abbreviations: SD (Standard Deviation); Min (Minimum value); Max (Maximum value); Sig (Significance).

Table 6: Values of the angles studied

Angle	Case 1	Case 2	Case 3	Case 5	Case 6	Case 8	Case 9	NV
1MDA	33.47º	37.25º	30.45º	21.07º	35.43º	31.07º	28.85º	23º
2MDA	28.83º	30.78º	28.57º	19.22º	23.91º	26.31º	26.17º	25º
5MDA	15.77º	14.12º	6.78º	9.14º	20.20º	12.98º	11.42º	15º
BA	23.34º	20.67º	36.65º	31.45º	29.26º	20.11º	36.67º	28-40º
CIA	25.86º	26.02º	20.15º	21.97º	26.27º	25.60º	21.92º	18-23º
FL	14.41º	24.20º	27.24º	9.60º	19.53º	20.79º	23.31º	0º
CAG	98.92º	107.07º	108.3º	116.36º	115.21º	106.75º	105.04º	120-145º
HA	134.81º	130.31º	140.02º	154.70º	138.10º	137.61º	138.57º	130º
MA	31.55º	25.41º	21.30º	9.75º	26.67º	21.79º	24.57º	0-14º
I-MCB	119.77º	105.88º	115.53º	130.49º	105.69º	114.47º	114.60º	115º
E-MCB	138.21º	137.79º	147.81º	140.60º	130.47º	138.8º	140.19º	145º
NH	4.32cm	3.49cm	3.79cm	3.14cm	4.36cm	3.33cm	3.79cm	3cm
PA	95.53º	93.82º	82.16º	92.86º	107.43º	97.50º	89.75º	81-95º
TDA	12.81º	11.40º	6.31º	14.03º	6.79º	8.07º	2.02º	25º
TCA	34.60º	36.32º	27.87º	32.14º	33.08º	32.71º	29.11º	35-40º
TTA	82.53º	82.88º	86.29º	68.28º	66.45º	74.79º	91.13º	60-77º

Abbreviations: NV (Normal Value).

Table 7: Normal variants and pathologies detected

	Case 1	Case 2	Case 3	Case 5	Case 6	Case 8	Case 9
Normal Variants							
Partial Fusion					+		
StiedaProcess	+	+			+		
Pathologies							
Bone Deformation				+			
Coalition		+					
Consolidated Fracture					+		
Fascia Calcification					+		
Spur			+		+		+
Haglund's Deformity	+	+		+	+		+
Osteoarthritis							
Cortical Degeneration	+	+	+	+	+		+
Osteophytes	+	+	+	+			+
Loss of Joint Space	+	+	+	+	+		+
Subchondral Sclerosis				+	+		+
Periostitis				+			

literature (Feix, 2000; Pettigrew, 1834; Dawson, 1927; Brier and Wade, 1997). These factors alter the composition of the muscles and bones, dehydrating and contracting them, as we observed in the mean of foot length (21.60cm, SD±2.27). Retraction is increased in the foot, but not in the leg. This may be due to the number of articulations in the foot, allowing it to be compacted much more than long bones such as the tibia and fibula.

Due to retraction, absence of toes and superimposition on the lateral projection, the toe formula was not possible to calculate. Yet, the metatarsal formula was calculated, with index minus being the most common in the population of the TT16. Due to the lack of dorso-plantar radiographies of the feet studied, the bone overlaying of the forefoot limited the correct differentiation of each bone, and the study of their morphology. Case 3 was the only one with dorso-plantar projection radiograph, where the talus head, metatarsals heads and first cuneiform morphology can be well described (FIGURE 7).

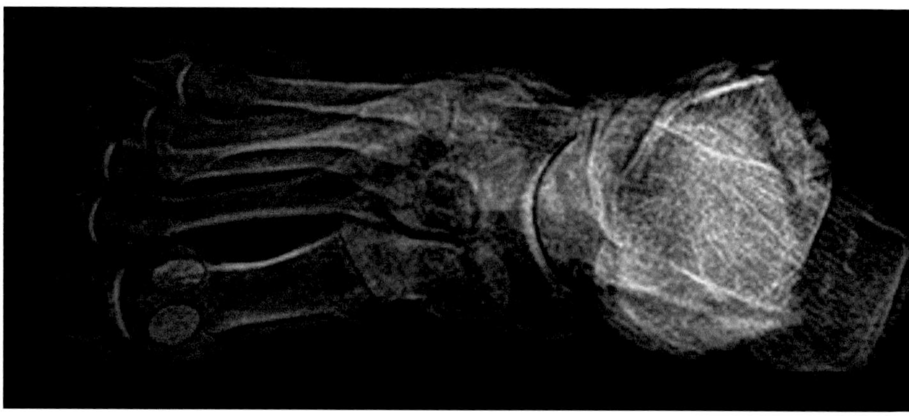

Figure 7.

Stature can play an important role in assessing environmental and social factors in past populations, including general health, sexual dimorphism and class differences Steegmann and Hasley, 1998). Trotter and Gleser's (Trotter and Glesser, 1958) formulae, based on long bone lengths for Black Americans has been used to estimate the stature of ancient Egyptians (Robins and Shute, 1983; Zakrzewski, 2003). However, many authors have postulated against using stature regression formulae derived from one population for others (Stevenson, 1929; Dupertuis and Hadden, 1951; Trotter and Gleser, 1952). According to these authors, Ratxer *et al.*, 2008 formulae was used in this study, and the results agree with the average height of general population in Third Intermediate Period calculated by Habicht *et al.* in 2015.

Age calculation was not exact as expected due to the lack of dorso-plantar radiographies of the feet. The absence of the secondary center of ossification of the calcaneus indicated no more than nine years in hypothetical male and seven in hypothetical female. However, the shape of the navicular and the talus indicated about 12 years in hypothetical male and nine in hypothetical female. Secondary centers of ossification on tibia and fibula indicated less than 12 years in hypothetical male and nine in hypothetical female (Hoerr *et al.*, 1962), settling the age approach.

Due to the lack of podiatry studies where angles of the foot and ankle in cadaver are calculated, the results obtained in the present study were compared with the values of normality accepted in the bibliography (Berquist, 2017; Christman, 2014; Montage, 1984). As expected, several angles have been statistically significant.

GA was altered, indicating calcaneal fracture, although this can be altered due to calcification changes over the time. Although two of the significant angles indicate pronation of the foot (TCA and HA), the alteration of most of them usually indicates the presence of a cavus foot in the living population. The augment of the NH, as well as the rupture of the FL and a positive value for the MA, indicate an increase of the plantar vault. Although the I-MCB has not been significant, MCB has, also indicating a cavus foot (Hetherington, 1994; Yalcin et al., 2010). The CIA indicates a medium cavus, while the 1MD can indicate both a cavus foot and a first plantarflexed radius. In addition, the alteration of the TTA indicates a forced flexed position of the TPA (Lamm *et al.*, 2016).

All of these significant values probably indicate an external pressure performed by the embalmers during mummification, while trying to recreate the normal shape of the foot, added to the retraction due to mummification. Natron and bandages were not the only agents that altered the morphology of the body. Subcutaneous body packing was a popular part of the embalming procedure, especially in the 21st dynasty (Smith and Dawson, 2002). The use of layers of mud in some regions of the human body was mainly for cosmetic reasons, to make the skin appear livelier. Therefore, it was important for the present study to make an accurate distinction between mummified soft tissue and embalming artifacts, such as corification and the presence of foreign bodies (Rühli and Böni, 2000)

Radiopathologic findings should be analysed with extreme caution because ancient remains may show conditions that are no longer present and known in present times. Most of the cases have a subchondral cut or fracture in which patella is missing. As there is no cortical reaction, the best explanation is that the limbs were separated from the post-mortem body, probably due to spoliation. The locations of the fractures (toes, ankle and knee) were typical areas where Egyptians placed amulets and jewellery (Salter-Pedersen, 2004).

Of the cases studied, case 8 was the only one that showed no signs of osteoarthritis, so it could be considered as a young adult with good quality of life. Spur (42.86%), fascia calcification (14.28%) and Haglund's deformity (57.14%), suggest muscle contraction and inextensibility in life (Berquist, 2017; Christman, 2014; Montage *et al.*, 1984). Incipient osteoarthritis was present in the 85.71% of the cases. Osteoarthritis is the most frequent joint disorder in the foot. It is not exclusive of the elderly population; in the foot and ankle, regardless of age, it is normally secondary to overuse and biomechanical abnormality of articulations (Berquist, 2017).

The present study has several limitations. Using a single evaluator for the radiographic measurements eliminated the potential for interevaluator bias. Also, because the lateral projection radiographs are not exactly lateral, at least some degree of measurement bias was present. Although the photomacrographic scale proved to be useful for this study, the lack or wrong placement of it could create some degree of measurement bias in approximate lengths and statures. The radiographies were collected in difficult conditions, and the lack of podiatric protocol for LE generated poor radiographic projections. Due to overlapping and lack of dorso-plantar radiograph, the midfoot and forefoot bones were difficult to isolate, especially the phalanges, which could not be assessed.

Superimposition in cases four and seven, due to the fact that the two legs were wrapped together, and the projections were not correct for their study, produced inaccurate results. Dorso-plantar projections of the foot have proved to be useful in bone identification and morphological study and it could help in angulometric studies. To remedy this in future lines of research, a radiology protocol for mummified lower extremities has been carried out.

Conclusions

A thorough knowledge of the foot structure is essential for an adequate interpretation of x-ray images of mummified lower extremities. A well-developed protocol can help the technicians who make the photographs and the x-rays in the field to do so in an adequate way for an accurate and exhaustive study. Hereby, podiatry can provide its experience to the paleontological study of human lower extremities, assessing foot pathologies and studying the behaviour of the foot structure due to the physical changes of the mummification process.

More studies need to be done to be able to affirm that the bandage and the natron retract the structures of the foot. Nevertheless, the present study can give an initial idea of this behaviour. It has been observed that the foot retracts in a cavus position, a foot type that could make the walk towards Aaru really uncomfortable.

Acknowlegements

First and foremost, thank the 'PROYECTO PANHESI TT16, LUXOR, EGIPTO', for the opportunity to collaborate in the project. Also, Dr Martínez-Escauriaza Peral, and Dra Dinarès Solà, for all their help in the elaboration of this study.

Bibliography

Berquist, T.H. 2017. Radiología de Pie y Tobillo. Madrid: Marban. 535.

Betrò, M. Del Vesco, P. Minaici, G. 2009. Seven seasons at Dra Abu El-Naga. The tomb of Huy (TT 14): preliminary results. Vol. 3. Pisa: Pisa University Press. 246.

Brier, B. Wade, R.S. 1997. The Use of Natron in Human Mummification: A Modern Experiment. Zeitschrift für Ägyptische Sprache und Altertumskunde. 124(2):89–100.

Christman, R. 2014. Foot and Ankle Radiology. 2nd edition. Philadelphia: LWW. 624.

Dawson, W.R. 1927. Making a Mummy. The Journal of Egyptian Archaeology. 13(1):40–9.

Dupertuis, C.W. Hadden, J.A. 1951. On the reconstruction of stature from long bones. American Journal of Physical Anthropology. 9(1):15–54.

El-Kilany, E. 2017. Foot Care: Uncommon Scenes in Ancient Egypt. International Journal of Heritage, Tourism, and Hospitality.

Feix, J. 2000. Herodot: Historien 1/2. Zweisprachige Ausgabe: GriechischDeutsch. Düsseldorf: Artemis and Winkler. 22.

Habicht, M.E. Henneberg, M. Öhrström, L.M. Staub, K. Rühli, F.J. 2015. Body height of mummified pharaohs supports historical suggestions of sibling marriages. American Journal of Physical Anthropology. 157(3):519–25.

Harpur, Y. Scremin, P. 2010. Egypt in miniature: The Chapel of Niankhkhnum and Khnumhotep. Scene Details. Martin GT, editor. Vol. 3. Oxford: Oxford University.

Hetherington, V. 1994. Hallux Valgus and Forefoot Surgery. New York: Churchill Livingstone. 599.

Hoerr, N.L. Pyle, S.I. Francis, C.C. 1962. Radiographic atlas of skeletal development of the foot and ankle: a standard of reference. Charles C. Thomas, editor. Springfield.

König, W. 1986. 14 Photographien mit Röntgenstrahlen. S.l.: Johann Ambrosius Barth.

Lamm, B. A. Stasko, P. Gesheff, M. Bhave, A. 2016. Normal Foot and Ankle Radiographic Angles, Measurements, and Reference Points. The Journal of foot and ankle surgery : official publication of the American College of Foot and Ankle Surgeons. 16;55.

Lynnerup, N. 2007. Mummies Yearbook. American Journal of Physical Anthropology. 134(45):162–90.

Montage, J. Chevrot, A. Galmiche, J.M. 1984. Atlas de Radiología del Pie. Masson editors. 1st edition. Madrid; 1984. ISBN 3431103477.

Pahl, W.M. Parsche, F. 1991. Unexplained findings in anthropologic study material from Egypt. Addenda to Herodotus' 'Historian', Lib. II, 86-88 and Egyptian 'Sparagmos'?. Anthropologischer Anzeiger. 49(1–2):39–48.

Panzer, S. Borumandi, F. Wanek, J. Papageorgopoulou, C. Shved, N. Colacicco, G. *et al.* 2013 'Modeling ancient Egyptian embalming': radiological assessment of experimentally mummified human tissue by CT and MRI. Skeletal Radiology. 42(11):1527–35.

Pettigrew, T.J. 1834. A history of Egyptian mummies, and an account of the worship and embalming of the sacred animals by the Egyptians; with remarks on the funeral ceremonies of different nations, and observations on the mummies of the Canary islands, of the ancient Peruvians, Burman priests, &c. London, Longman, Rees, Orme, Brown, Green and Longman. 328

Porter, B. Moss, R.L.B. 2004. Topographical Bibliography of Ancient Egyptian Hieroglyphic Texts, Statues, Reliefs and Paintings. Volume I Part 1. The Theban Necropolis. Private Tombs. Malek J, editor. 2nd edition. Oxford: Griffith Institute; ISBN 0900416 815.

Raxter, M.H. Ruff, C.B. Azab, A. Erfan, M. Soliman, M. El-Sawaf, A. 2008. Stature estimation in ancient Egyptians: a new technique based on anatomical reconstruction of stature. American Journal of Physical Anthropology.136(2):147–55.

Robins, G. Shute, C.C.D. 1983. The physical proportions and living stature of New Kingdom pharaohs. Journal of Human Evolution. 12: 455–465

Rühli, F.J. 1998. Paläopathologische Untersuchungen an einer altägyptischen Mumie aus den Naturwissenschaftlichen Sammlungen der StadtWinterthur. Zürich? Dietikon. 299.

Rühli, F.J. Chhem, R.K. Böni, T. 2004. Diagnostic paleoradiology of mummified tissue: interpretation and pitfalls. Canadian Association of Radiologists Journal. 55(4):218–27.

Rühli, F.J. Böni, T. 2000. Radiological aspects and interpretation of post-mortem artefacts in ancient Egyptian mummies from Swiss collections. International Journal of Osteoarchaeology. 10(2):153–7.

Salter-Pedersen, E. 2004. The myth of eternal preservation: patterns of damage in Egyptian mummies. [Internet thesis]. [Louisiana]: Louisiana State University and Agricultural and Mechanical College; 2004 [cited 2018 May 24]. Available from: https://digitalcommons.lsu.edu/cgi/viewcontent.cgi?article=1966&context=gradschool_theses

Sluglett, J. 1990. Mummification in Ancient Egypt. The West England Medical Journal. Dec;105(4):117–9.

Smith GE, Dawson WR. 2002. Egyptian mummies. London : Kegan Paul.

Steegmann, A.T. Hasely, P.A. 1988. Stature variation in the British American colonies: French and Indian War records, 1755–1763. American Journal of Physical Anthropology. 75:413–421.

Stevenson, P.H. 1929. On Racial Differences in Stature Long Bone Regression Formulae, with Special Reference to Stature Reconstruction Formulae for the Chinese. Biometrika. 21(1/4):303–21.

Trotter, M. Gleser, G.C. 1952. Estimation of stature from long bones of American Whites and Negroes. American Journal of Physical Anthropology. 10(4):463–514.

Trotter, M. Gleser, G.C. 1958. A re-evaluation of estimation of stature based on measurements of stature taken during life and of long bones after death. American Journal of Physical Anthropology. 16(1):79–123.

Yalcin, N. Esen, E. Kanatli, U. Yetkin, H. 2010. Evaluation of the medial longitudinal arch: A comparison between the dynamic plantar pressure measurement system and radiographic analysis. Acta orthopaedica et traumatologica turcica. 1;44:241–5.

Zakrzewski, S.R. 2003. Variation in ancient Egyptian stature and body proportions. American Journal of Physical Anthropology. 121:219–229.

Egyptian Medical Civilization: from Dawn of History to Kasr Al Ainy School

Sahar Saleem

Saharsaleem1@gmail.com
Kasr Al Ainy Faculty of Medicine-Cairo University, Cairo

Abstract: The science and art of medicine has always been an integral part of the history of Egypt. Medical practice in ancient Egypt was based on the most advanced knowledge compared to other regions. Muslim scholars helped in the transmission of medical practice through the medieval period from the decline of ancient teaching to the rise of modern learning. Kasr Al Ainy school of Medicine, established in 1827, continues the glory of medicine in Egypt as one of the biggest and oldest medical schools not only in Egypt but also in the world.

Keywords: medicine, ancient Egypt, Kasr Al Ainy, paleopathology, mummies

The glory of medicine in Egypt in ancient world

The science and medical knowledge was advanced in Egypt compared to neighbouring nations during ancient times. Patients from other countries sought the help of Egyptian physicians, who were held in high regard, to treat their ailments. The Persian King Cyrus requested the Egyptian King Ahmose II (26th dynasty, 560 BC) to send him the best Egyptian eye doctor (Nunn, 1996, p. 198)

Ancient Egyptian Physicians

There is a long list of legendary physicians in ancient Egypt that includes:

Imhotep (2667 BC-2648 BC) the true father of medicine who treated more than 200 diseases, a multi-talented vizier of King Djoser (3rd dynasty) and the architect who designed the first stone pyramid (Saqqara). Imhotep was elevated to the status of a full God in later dynasties and was equated by the Greeks with Asklepios, the Greek god of Medicine (Luth, 1963, p.p. 826-827) (Figure 1).

Hesy ra (3rd Dynasty-contemporary of Imhotep) was the first person in history to have the professional title of 'dentist' (Nunn, 1996, p. 124).

Peseshet (5th Dynasty): A female physician and overseer of female physicians. (Nunn, 1996, p. 124).

Medical specialities

Herodotus, the Greek historian (484-425 BC) wrote about specialization in the medical practice in ancient Egypt: 'The practice of medicine is so divided among them that each physician treats one disease, and no more. There are plenty of physicians everywhere, some are eye-doctors, some deal with the head, others with the teeth or the belly, and some with hidden maladies' (Todd, 1921, p. 462).

Hierarchy of physicians

There were ranks of physicians in ancient Egypt: regular physician (swnw), senior physician, chief physician, overseer of physicians, inspector of physicians, and court physician (doctor of the royal family) (Nunn, 1996, p. 117).

Advanced medical practice

Medical practice in ancient Egypt was so advanced that it included:

- Medical insurance: Physicians were appointed by the state for treating every citizen.
- Occupational medicine: A physician was appointed in workers' camps to look after their health and treat occupational injuries (physician Perhipidje worked at Deir el Medina, the campus of tomb builders in Luxor) (Nunn, 1996, p. 75).
- Military medicine: An inscription of the Battle of Kadesh (1274 BC) shows a man (physician) attending to the leg of a soldier. (Nunn, 1996, p. 121).

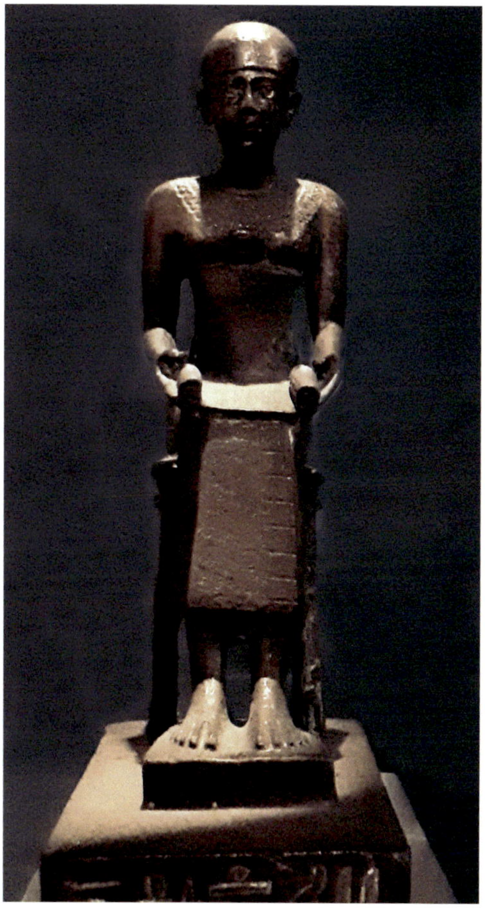

Figure 1: Statue of Imhotep, the true father of medicine (2667 BC-2648 BC) displayed at 'Imhotep Museum' in Saqqara- Egypt
The statue shows Imhotep seated with his hands resting on his knees holding a papyrus roll on his lap

Medical Education in ancient Egypt

Advanced medical specialization and hierarchy of physicians in ancient Egypt, were a reflection of the advanced medical education that took place at institutes called 'Peri-ankh' or 'the Houses of Life' (Gardiner 1938, p.p. 157-179). The first medical institution opened in the first dynasty (3150-2925 BC) and many others followed across the land of Egypt. In the north of Egypt, the House of Life at Sais was famous for its female faculty physicians instructing female physicians and midwives. Peseshet (c. 2500 BC) was 'overseer of female physicians' at school of Sais as well the personal doctor of the royal palace. She is cited as the world's first known female physician (Harer and el-Dawakhly, 1989, p. 960).

Medical information in ancient Egypt was written in papyri according to the specialization to serve as references for physicians. The most famous were Edwin Smith (copied in 1600 BC from an original text dated to the 1st dynasty 3000 BC), concerned with surgery; Ebers Papyrus (3000 BC) dealt with the treatment of women and children; Kahun papyrus (1825 BC) dealt with internal medicine. The medical information in these papyri discussed clinical cases in the same steps we follow in our modern medical education books. The physician interrogated the patient about their medical history then performed systematic clinical examinations of the body that included inspection, palpation and percussion. This was followed by a diagnosis, prognosis (treatable or not), then treatment, if appropriate. Most of the cases included explanatory notes for unfamiliar terms and clarification of the descriptions (Nunn, 1996, p.p. 25-35).

Timeline of medical practice from ancient Egypt to modern times through the Middle Ages

Medical practice in Egypt was widely respected among other nations. The greatest of Greek physicians, Hippocrates (ca 460BC-370BC), Herophilos (ca335-280 BC), Erasistratus (ca 310 BC-250BC, and Galen (ca 130 AD-210 AD) all studied in Egypt and acknowledged the contribution of Egyptian medicine to Greek medicine (Hall, 2014, p.p. 20-30). The ancient library of Alexandria (c. 288 BC) was the centre of knowledge in the ancient world; its 700,000 scrolls attracted many scholars and physicians from all over the world (Serageldin, 2013, p.p. 395-404). However in several aspects, the medical knowledge of Egyptians surpassed that of Greek physicians, such as Hippocrates and Galen, who lived over 1000 years later (Hall, 2014, p.p. 20-30).

The decline of the ancient Egyptian medical civilization was triggered by the Persian occupation of Egypt (525 BCE) which targeted and destroyed the Egyptian medical institutes (Peri-Ankh). Medical civilization in Egypt declined slowly due to being recurrently occupied by several foreign nations [Serageldin, 2013, p.p. 395-404).

In Medieval times, medicine in Egypt was influenced by the famous Muslim physicians Al-Razi (864-930 AD) and Avicenna (980-1037 AD). Those scholars helped in the transmission of medical practice throughout the dark ages, from the decline of ancient teaching to the rise of modern learning (Browne, 2002, p.p. 1-138). The hospital was one of the greatest achievements of medieval Islamic society. The medieval Islamic hospital was a more elaborate institution with a wider range of functions than the earlier sick relief facilities offered by some Christian monasteries in Egypt. Some hospitals were medical teaching institutions with formal classes and bedside clinical training (Dols and Adil, 1984, p. 6).

During the Turkish occupation in the 16th century, medical practice in Egypt declined considerably, a situation which lasted until Mohamed Ali Pasha ruled Egypt (1805-1848 AD). Concerned about the health of the army, Mohamed Ali Pasha appointed Antoine Barthelemy Clot, doctor of internal medicine and surgeon from Marseilles, to organize health services in Abu Zabel military hospital. To fulfill the army needs, Dr Clot proposed a teaching course to train Egyptian physicians (El-Minawi and Nuweisar, 2000.p.p. 26-28)

Foundation of Egypt's Medical School (Kasr Al Ainy 1827)

One hundred students were drawn from al-Azhar, the Islamic institute in Cairo, to study a five-year course of medical training designed by Clot. An introductory year to mathematics and science was followed by four-year medical curriculum. The first year included the study of anatomy, pathology, and material medica. The second year included physiology, surgery, and therapeutics. The third and fourth years were clinical training in internal medicine and surgery in addition to hygiene, toxicology and forensic medicine. Postmortem dissection was a

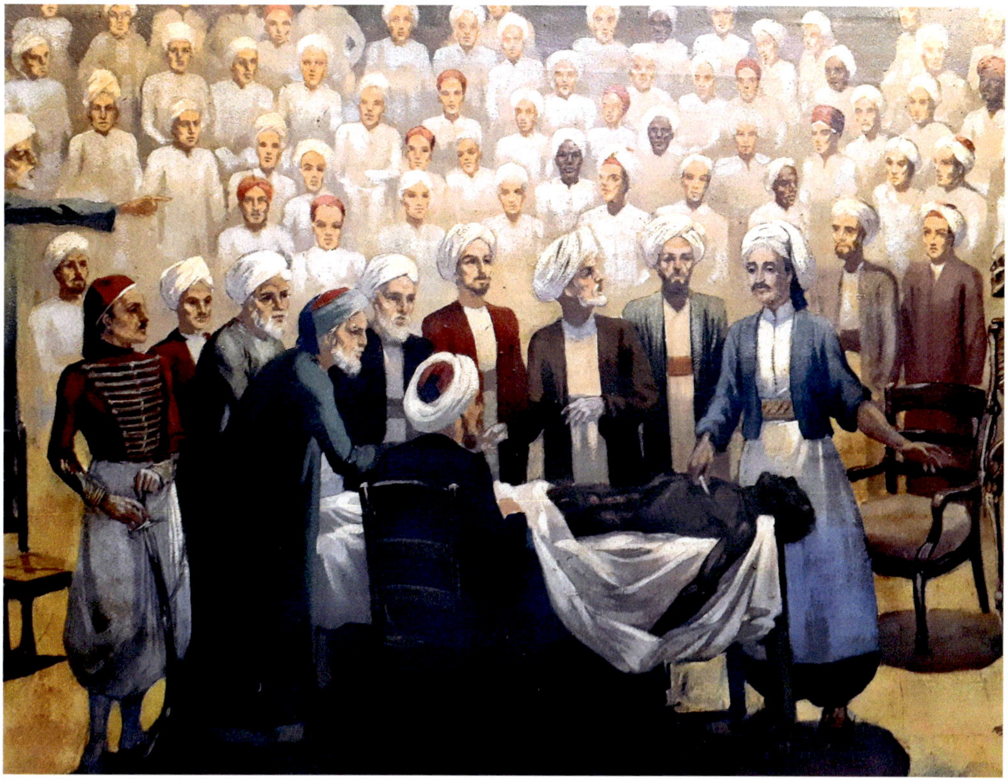

Figure 2: Dissection Class at 'Kasr Al Ainy School of Medicine' 1837
Oil painting displayed at Kasr Al Ainy School of Medicine Museum shows Dr Clot, the director of Kasr Al Ainy School, in a practical dissection lesson of a human corpse in front of the students and 'sheikhs', Muslim religious figures

regular teaching routine despite the resistance of some students and Muslim religious figures (shaykhs) (Figure 2) (Kuhnke, 1990, p.35).

Clot was the director of the School and taught surgery. Faculty staff members were Europeans who needed interpreters for Arabic. The class was divided into ten groups; each group had ten students led by the smartest among them who coached every member of his group. Foreign visitors thought that this student mentoring system was a European invention, but in fact this had been the tutorial system of al-Azhar Islamic institute, the students' former school, for centuries (Kuhnke, 1990, p.35).

Egyptian faculty members of the school: Twelve graduates of class year 1832 were sent to Paris to study for doctorates in six different specializations and thus to form the nucleus of the Egyptian teaching staff in natural history, physics and chemistry, pharmacy, anatomy and physiology, pathology, internal medicine, and surgery (El-Minawi and Nuweisar, 2000, p.p. 29-30) (Figure 3).

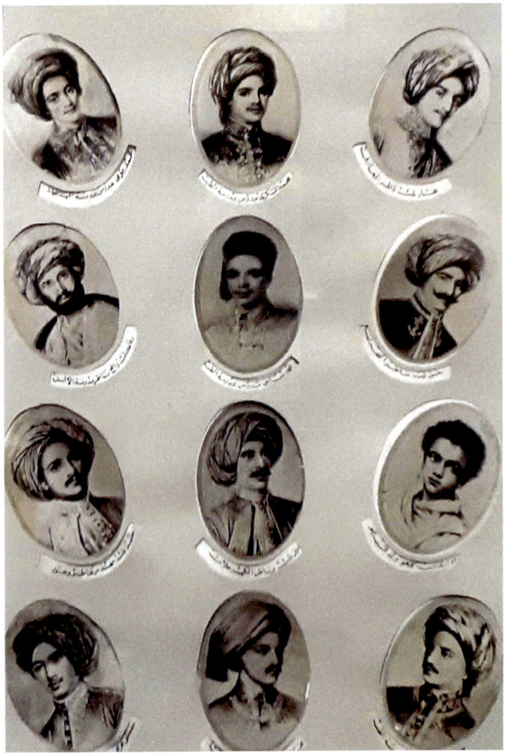

Figure 3: First class graduates of 'Kasr Al Ainy School of Medicine' year 1832

Medical Education programs at Kasr Al Ainy

In 1837, the school of Medicine and hospital were transferred from Abu Zabal to a building on the bank of the River Nile (Kasr Al Ainy palace founded in 1466). (El-Minawi and Nuweisar, 2000, p.p. 29-30).

Medical Education at Kasr Al Ainy (19th century-early 20th century)

With the inclusion of Egyptians as instructors, all courses were conducted in Arabic after 1839. The first Egyptian director of Kasr Al Ainy School of Medicine was Dr. Mohamad El-Sahfei in year 1847.

By the year 1849, 55 textbooks were translated to Arabic. Graduates of Kasr Al Ainy medical school mastered not only their medical knowledge and training, but also foreign languages (French), and contributed in research studies. Arabic remained the language of teaching at Kasr Al Ainy till 1880s, when the British occupation transferred the studies from Arabic to English language. Since that time, studies have been in English at Kasr Al Ainy Faculty of Medicine (El-Minawi and Nuweisar, 2000, p. 31).

The first International Conference on Medicine was held at Kasr Al Ainy in December 1902 with the participation of physicians from America, Britain, France, Italy, Swiss, Spain, Germany, and Austria.

In October 1926, the School was transferred to a Faculty associated with the Egyptian University (Cairo University).

In 1927, the foundation of the 'new' building of Kasr Al Ainy school of medicine was laid across the river Nile, parallel to the old school; the old and new buildings have been connected by two bridges.

Since then, Kasr Al Ainy Medical School has established its status and attracted students from all over the Arab world, spreading medical practices in the region (El-Dib, 2015, p.p. 1-7).

Featured Activities of Kasr Al Ainy School of Medicine (19th century to early 20th century)

Defeating Small Pox:

Antoine Colt (1793-1868)

The early part of the 19th century witnessed smallpox outbreaks that killed 60,000 in Egypt each year. In 1819, the Egyptian government initiated a smallpox eradication program that extended till1850. Physicians were sent to the countryside to vaccinate children and to instruct local barbers in the techniques to continue the program. Since opening in 1827, the Egyptian medical school 'Kasr Al Ainy' participated in the government's nationwide smallpox immunization program (Figure 4). The director of the School, Dr Clot, prepared a detailed instruction on the technique and signs that indicated successful vaccination. In 1856, the immunization center for children opened at Kasr Al Ainy School of Medicine, enabling the defeat of smallpox. By the end of the 19th century Egypt was comparatively free from smallpox (Kuhnke 1990, p.p. 35-133).

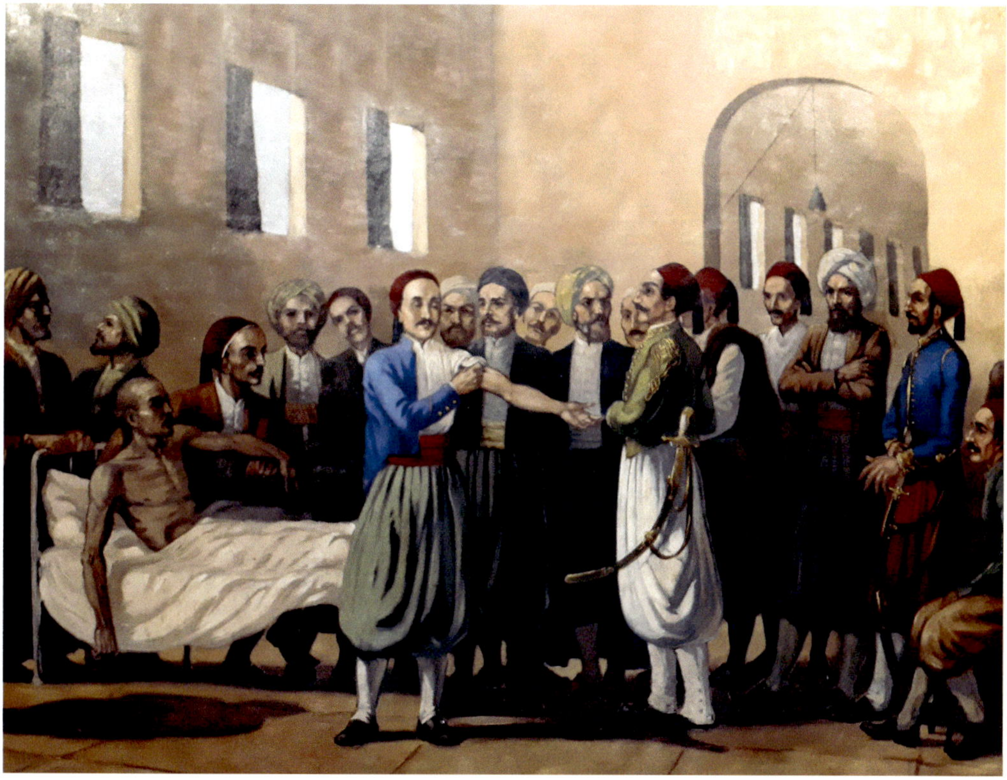

Figure 4: Small Pox vaccination 1835
Oil painting displayed at Kasr Al Ainy School of Medicine Museum shows Dr Clot, the director of Kasr Al Ainy School, demonstrating the technique of smallpox vaccination by inoculating himself with pus from a plague bubo. Kasr Al Ainy School of Medicine had important role in eradication of small pox in Egypt

Discovery of Schistosomiasis:

Theodor Maximilian Bilharz (1825-1862)

The German professor Theodor Bilharz was born in Sigmaringen in 1825 and studied medicine at Tübingen University. In 1849 he passed the state examination, and in 1850 he received his Doctorate.

In 1850, Bilharz was appointed as an assistant to professor Wilhelm Griesinger, Chief of Health and Supervisor or Kasr Al Ainy School of Medicine in Cairo (Figure 5).

In 1852, Bilharz was offered a Professorship of Anatomy at Kasr Al Ainy School of Medicine. In 1853 Bilharz identified the parasite causing severe illness since ancient Egyptian times and named it 'Distomum haematobium'. Later, in 1984, the International commission on Zoological Nomenclature adopted the name Schistosoma for the parasite, and the disease was named Bilharziasis after his name.

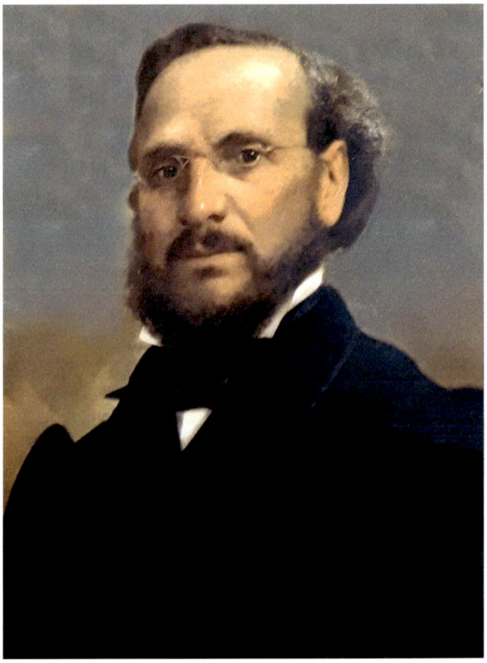

Figure 5: Theodor Bilharz (1825-1862)
Oil painting of Theodor Bilharz portrait displayed at Kasr Al Ainy School of Medicine Museum. Bilharz worked as assistant professor of bacteriology then professor of anatomy at Kasr Al Ainy School of Medicine (1850-1862)

During his work at Kasr Al Ainy School of Medicine, Bilharz also discovered *Heterophyes heterophyes*, and described the electrical organ of the thunder fish.

Bilharz was fond of Egypt. He started learning the Arabic language and hieroglyphics. His hand drawings of Egyptian birds are displayed at Kasr Al Ainy school of Medicine Museum (El Dib, 2019, p.p. 3-6)

During a hunting expedition in Somalia in 1862, Bilharz caught a fatal disease (typhoid or typhus). He died a few days after he returned to Cairo, where he was buried. Egypt honoured the memory of Bilharz by establishing a research Institute that was named after him (Theodor Bilharz). A statue of Bilharz is still at the department of parasitology in Kasr Al Ainy school of medicine, and his hand drawings are exhibited at the museum of Kasr Al Ainy. In addition, the government issued a postal stamp with Bilharz photo in 1962 (Eltawil, and Plassmann M., 2011, p.p. 17-25)

Mummy studies and the foundation of paleopathology at Kasr Al Ainy

The massive excavations that took place in Egypt in the 19th century unearthed thousands of mummies. Many of those mummies were sent to Kasr Al Ainy medical school to be examined by the school's professors. The museum of the Anatomy Department at Kasr Al Ainy in fact still hosts mummies and displays ancient Egyptian human remains (Figure 6).

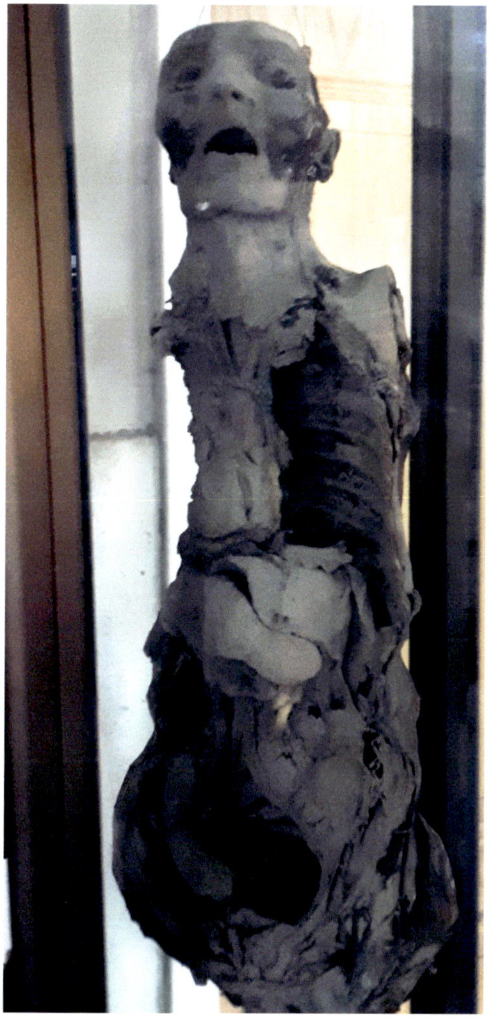

Figure 6a: Mummified human body at the Anatomy Museum in Kasr Al Ainy School of Medicine. Ancient Egyptians mummies unearthed during excavations in the 19th century were sent to be studied at Kasr Al Ainy School of Medicine.

Kasr Al Ainy School of Medicine thus gave a golden opportunity to several professors to start, practice, and be pioneers in mummy studies. Smith, Derry, and Ruffer are among this list (Harris, 1998, p. 59) (Figure 7).

Sir Grafton Eliot Smith *(1871-1937):*

Elliot Smith was born in Grafton, New South Wales. In 1883, the family moved to Sydney. In 1888, Smith started his medical studies at University of Sydney and graduated in 1895. In 1896, Smith went to England and joined St John's College, Cambridge. From 1900 to 1909, Smith was appointed professor then head of the Anatomy department of Kasr Al Ainy Medical School. In 1901, Smith was consulted on anatomical data of ancient Egyptian remains. During his work at Kasr Al Ainy, Smith unwrapped and examined thousands of ancient Egyptian mummies and skeletons (Blunt, 1988, p. 11).

Smith was one of the first scholars to study Egyptian mummies using radiological techniques. In 1903, Smith with the help of the Egyptian radiologist El-Khayat studied by x-ray the mummy of king Ramesses IV (1155-1149 BC). The mummy of king Ramesses IV was taken on a horse-driven taxi to a medical facility with an x-ray machine. Smith also examined most of the royal mummies at the Egyptian museum in Cairo. He published the findings of anatomical examination of the royal mummies in a monograph (Smith, 1912, p.p. 1-92), and with Warren Dawson in a book (Smith and Dawson, 1924, p.p. 1-30). Smith also studied the mummies in Nubia (Waldron, 2000, p.p.363-388).

Smith returned to England in 1909. He worked as Professor of Anatomy in Manchester (1909-1919) then Chair of Anatomy at University College London (1919-1937). Smith stayed in a nursing home in London in the last year of his life and died on first day of 1937 (Blunt, 1988, p. 11).

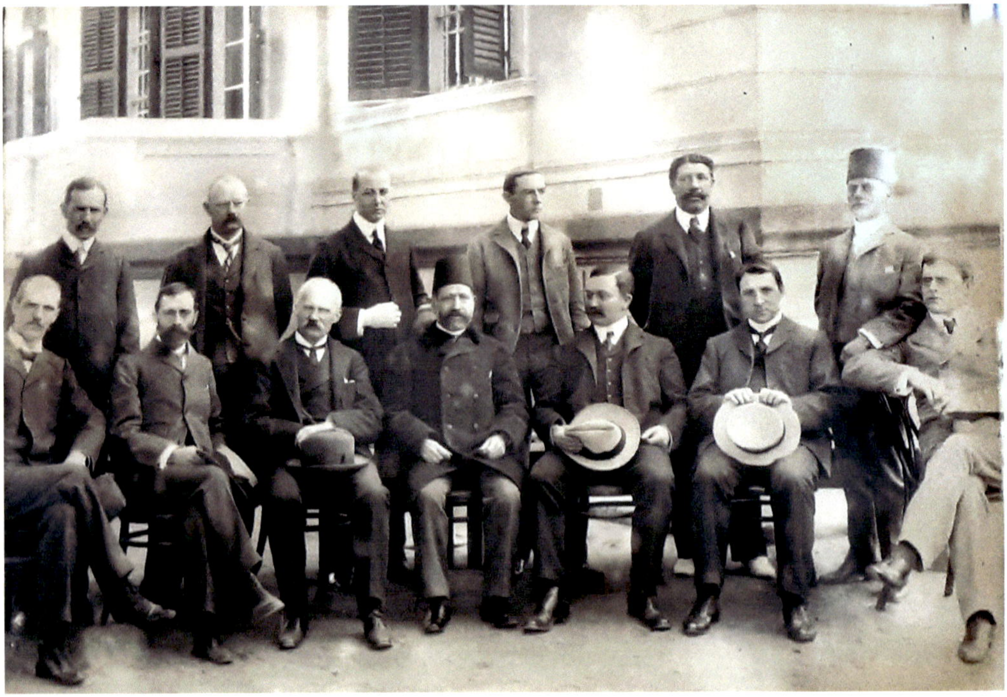

Figure 7: A photograph of the Professors of Kasr Al Ainy School of Medicine (from 1890-1903). Standing from left to right: Dr Elliot Smith (anatomy), Dr Arthur Looss (parasitology), Dr Trabib (Genera; medicine), Dr Nolen (Forensic), Dr Mohamad Shokry (Obstetrics and gynecology), Fisher (ophthalmology). Sitting from left to right: Schmidt (Chemistry), William Hawkins Wilson (physiology), FM Sandwith (General medicine), Ibrahim Hassan (Dean), Keatinge (director), Francis Cole Madden (surgery), and Symmers (pathology)

Douglas Erith Derry (1874-1961)

Douglas Derry studied medicine in Edinburgh. Following his graduation in 1903, Derry worked in the Department of Anatomy in Edinburgh.

In 1905, Derry was appointed as Assistant Professor in the Anatomy department of Kasr Al Ainy and held this position for about thirty years. Beside his academic work, Derry assisted in the archeological work in Nubia mainly by taking bone measurements.

In 1919, Derry was appointed as the head of the Anatomy Department. This post at Kasr Al Ainy gave Derry a great opportunity to be the first anatomist to examine the mummy of king Tutankhamun (1341-1323 BC) together with Dr Saleh Bey Hamdi, an Egyptian physician (Fielding, 1961, p.p. 441-442).

Sir Marc Armand Ruffer (1859-1917)

Ruffer was born in Lyons in France in 1859. He graduated in medicine at London, and studied at Pasteur Institute. In 1891 Ruffer became the first director of the British Institute of Preventive Medicine. During his studies on diphtheria, Ruffer caught an infection and was paralyzed.

He resigned and left to Egypt for rehabilitation. Ruffer was appointed then at Kasr Al Ainy Medical School as a professor of Bacteriology. He helped in the eradication of cholera in Egypt. (Sandison, 1967, p.p. 150-156).

Ruffer joined the flourishing mummy studies program at Kasr Al Ainy. He was the first to find calcified schistosoma egg in two ancient Egyptian mummies of the 20th Dynasty (1250-1000 BC) (Ruffer, 1910, p.16) and arterial atherosclerosis in mummies dating from the 18th Dynasty (1550 BC-1298 BC) to the Coptic period (3rd-4th centuries AD) (Ruffer, 1911, p.p.453-462)..

In 1910, Elliot Smith and Ruffer identified tuberculosis of the spine (Pott's disease) in a mummy of the 20th dynasty; the diagnosis was based on bony affection as well as a large psoas abscess in the preserved soft tissue (Smith and Ruffer, 1910, p. 3)

A year earlier, their colleague Douglas Derry suggested tuberculosis in ancient Egyptian skeletal remains but based only on bony changes (Derry, 1983, p.p. 196-199).

Modern medical practice at Kasr Al Ainy Faculty of Medicine passing to 2019

Nowadays, Kasr Al Ainy comprises of a complex of specialized hospitals with a total capacity of about 5000 beds serving about two million patients a year. Thirty four medical departments belong to the school, namely: anatomy, histology, biochemistry, microbiology, pharmacology, parasitology, forensic, public health, ophthalmology, urology, neurology, rheumatology, orthopedics, cardiology, oncology, pediatrics, anesthesia, obstetrics and gynecology, internal medicine, endemic medicine, general surgery, plastic surgery, neurosurgery, pulmonary medicine, dermatology, andrology, cardiothoracic surgery, family medicine, critical care, psychological medicine, ear nose and throat, dermatology, oncology, and radiology (Kasr Al Ainy, 2019).

The hierarchy of faculty members at Kasr Al Ainy Faculty of medicine matches those at other modern medical institutes. The hierarchy includes the dean, heads of medical departments, professors, other attending physicians, fellows, and residents. The minister of health is the physician leader who overseas all medical facilities and establishes policies and practice.

Medical, academic and scientific activities:

Kasr Al Ainy School of medicine offers education programs for undergraduate and postgraduate students. The students come from Egypt as well as from several countries such as Iraq, Yemen, Libya, Malaysia, Nepal, and more. The medical programs at Kasr Al Ainy provide the students with adequate knowledge and competent clinical experience to serve in medical care of their societies.

Kasr Al Ainy also prepares the students to be scholars and to be able to conduct research work. Many research studies and trials are carried in Kasr Al Ainy school of medicine every year, the results of which are published in prestigious medical journals and scientific publications.

In modern history, Kasr Al Ainy Faculty of medicine continues the glory of medicine in Egypt. As the testimony of Paul Ghalioungi (1908-1987), Egyptian physician graduate of Kasr Al Ainy (1929), PhD internal medicine (1933), and author, relates: 'The institution of healing in ancient Egypt was as much organized in ancient Egypt as it is today' (Ghalioungui, 1973, p.p, 1-19)

And in the testimony of the author of this article: 'We were never far from where we are'.

References

Breasted, JH (1930) The Edwin Smith Surgical papyrus. Chicago: University of Chicago Press

Browne, E.G. (2001) Islamic medicine. New Delhi: Goodword books

Derry, D.E. (1938), Pott's disease in ancient Egypt, Med. Press 1

Dols, M.W. and Adil S.G. (1984) Medieval Islamic medicine: Ibn Ridwan's treatise 'On the prevention of bodily ills in Egypt. Berkeley: University of California Press

El Dib, N.A. (2015) 'Kasr Al Ainy, the story of a palace that became a medical school', Kasr Al Ainy Med J, 21

El-Minawi, M.F. and Nuweisar H.M. (2000) The renaissance of Egyptian medical history. Cairo: Nahdet Misr

Eltawil, K.M. and Plassmann, M. (2011)'Theodor Maximilian Bilharz (1825-1862)', International Journal of Parasitology Research, 3(1)

Fielding, R. (1961). 'Douglas Erith Derry', J. Anat., 95(3)

Gardiner, A.H. (1938) 'The House of Life', The Journal of Egyptian Archaeology, 24(1)

Ghalioungi, P. (1973), The house of life: Per ankh, magic and medical science in ancient Egyp, Amesterdam: B.M. Israel

Hajar, R. (2012) 'The Air of History: Early Medicine to Galen', Heart Views, 13(3)

Hall, T. (2014) History of Medicine: All that matters. London: Hachette

Harer, W.B. and el-Dawakhly, Z. 'Peseshet-the first female physican?', Obstet Gynecol, 74, p.p.960-1

Harris J.E., Pontiz P.V., Ingalls B.K. Dental health in ancient Egypt. In Mummies, diseases, and ancient cultures. Ed. Cockburn E., Cockburn A., Reyman T.A. Cambridge Cambridge University Press

Kasr Al Ainy (2019) Organization Chart http://www.medicine.cu.edu.eg/index.php/en/departments (accessed Sept 3, 2019)

Kuhnke, L (1990) Lives at Risk: Public Health in Nineteenth Century Egypt. Berleley: University of California Press

Luth, V.P. (1963) ' Imhotep Oder Asklepios: On the beginning of scientific medicine in Egypt and Greece'. Hippocrate, 34

Nunn, JF (1996) Ancient Egyptian Medicine. Norman: University of Oklahoma Press

Ruffer, M.A. (1910). 'Note on the present of Bilharzia haematobia in Egyptian mummies of the 20th dynasty (1250-1000 B.C'. Journal of Pathology and Bacteriology

Saleem, S.N., Sabri, Y.Y (2012) Measuring competence of Radiology Education Programs and Residents: The Egyptian Experience. In Radiology Education: The Evaluation and Assessment of Clinical Competence. Berlin Heidelberg: Springer-Verlag

Sandison, A.T. (1967) 'Sir Marc Armand Ruffer (1859-1917) pioneer of paleopathology' Med Hist, 11(2)

Serageldin, I. (2013) 'Ancient Alexandria and the dawn of medical science', Glob Cardiol Sci Pract, 4

Smith, G.E. (1912) The royal mummies, Catalogue General du Musee du Caire, Nos 61051-61100, Cairo (http://www.cesras.org/Smith-CG-Royal-Mummies/03SmithIndex.html)

Smith, G.E. and Dawson W.R. (1924) Egyptian mummies. London: George Alen and Unwin

Smith, G.E., and Ruffer, M.A. (1910) . 'Pott'sche Krankheit an einer Agyptschen mumie aus der Zeit der 21 Dynastie (Um 1000 V.Chr.)' in Zur historischen Biologie der Krankheits erreger, ed. Sudhoff und Sticker, Heft 3, Giessen

Sonbol A. (1991) The creation of medical profession in Egypt, 1800-1922. Syracuse, NY: Syracuse University Press

Todd, T. (1921). Egyptian Medicine: A Critical Study of Recent Claims. American Anthropologist, 23(4), new series, 460-470.

Waldron, H. A (2000) 'The study of the human remains from Nubia: the contribution of Grafton Elliot Smith and his colleagues to paleopathology'. *Med Hits, 44(3) at* https://www.ncbi.nlm.nih.gov/pmc/articles/PMC1044289/?page=3

The Pure Priest of Sekhmet, Between Health and Disease

Núria Torras Benezet

nuria.torras@ub.edu
University of Barcelona

Abstract: In addition to his particular skill and knowledge in calming the goddess Sekhmet, the *wab*-priest had other functions and abilities. In the sources we find him described both as an expert in making medical diagnoses by observing blood circulation and as the veterinarian responsible for the bull stables in the temples. He was the only one with the ability to distinguish the living hypostases of the god Apis and was enabled to certify the purity of the animals to be sacrificed. By the ritual slaughter and butchering of bulls under his supervision the prophylactic protection of Egypt was sought.

However, the *wab*-priest of Sekhmet had a double role: he spread diseases and also cured them. This duality defined the priest as much as it defined the ambivalent goddess he served. Indeed, holding life and death in her hands, this goddess had the privilege of preserving life as well as the power to send calamities. The *wab*-priest could interact with Sekhmet since his purity immunized him from the dangerous effects of the goddess' fury. Once she had been pacified and ritually neutralized, Sekhmet's qualities were transferred to and assimilated by her officiant. The survival of these officiants into the Roman period is further proof of the cultural resilience of Ancient Egypt under Greco-Roman domination.

Keywords: *wab*-priest, medical diagnosis, purity, Sekhmet, Apis, animal sacrifice, double *was*-sceptre province, *moschosphragistēs*.

Introduction

The pure (*wab*) priest of the goddess Sekhmet was a type of ancient Egyptian ritualist closely linked to the Houses of Life that played an important role in the protection of the country, the living image of Apis and the practice of medicine. They were considered magicians of a high intellectual level and normally held a high social status (Torras 2017a: 16).

The pure priests of the goddess Sekhmet often also served in temples as priest-readers –*ẖry-ḥb ḥry-tp*–, as we can see from the statue of Iuny and his wife Renenutet found in Amenhotep's tomb chapel in Asyut. The list of all his titles on the base of the statue tells us that Iuny was a priest-reader, head of the pure priests of Sekhmet and son of Amenhotep, who held the same post.

The title of 'head of the pure priests of Sekhmet' could be inherited and was frequently passed down from father to son or from uncle to nephew. On the Naples stela, Darius III accords Somtoutefnekht:

> '(...) il (le souverain d'Asie) érigea pour moi la fonction de directeur des prêtres-ouâb de Sekhmet, à la place du frère de ma mère, le dirécteur des prêtres-ouâb de Sekhmet de Haute et Basse Égypte, Nakhthéneb'.[1]

[1] Naples stela of *Sematawytefnakht* 1035 (Museo Archeologico Nazionale di Napoli), l.9-10 [Urk. II, 4, 1-2].Transl. Känel (1984: 121).

Pharmacy and Medicine in Ancient Egypt
(Archaeopress 2021): 116–124

Nakhtheneb was probably given the title of 'head of the pure priests of Sekhmet of Upper and Lower Egypt' in return for services to the Persian court, although this title of his is not previously documented. In the case of the nephew, Darius III granted him the highest rank given until then: 'head of the pure priests of Sekhmet of all the earth', of the entire civilized world (Känel 1984: 249).

The quick-tempered Sekhmet, who was served by this type of priest, personified the destructive power of the sun. However, once ritually appeased, the 'furious one who kills' became the 'satisfied one who gives life'. Once assuaged, she became a beneficent and protective entity who granted the king long years of renewed life and a prosperous reign, as well as protection against illness and enemies.

Holding life and death in her hands, she had the privilege of preserving life, as well as the power of sending calamities. The suffocating heat of the month of *Epiphi* (May-June), fevers, epidemics and the pollution of the waters of the Nile were considered to be acts of the goddess Sekhmet and her emissaries that preceded the annual arrival of the flood (Yoyotte 1980: 56-57).

All were vulnerable to her seven arrows, especially during the epagomenal days (additional days of the year). Even the spoiling of food was attributed to her short-tempered actions. A formula for purifying food offerings engraved in the Temple of Horus in Edfu [*Edfou* VI, 155, 8-12] asks her to provide healthy food for the table of the king and to direct her arrow to contaminate the food of 'those who shall speak any malicious word' against the pharaoh, in the sense of an incantation for evil purposes (Yoyotte 1980: 69, 75 n. 69).

The *wab*-priest was able to interact with this deity and assuage her, as his purity immunized him from the dangerous effects of her power. In addition to his skill and specific knowledge of how to appease the goddess Sekhmet, the *wab*-priest had other important functions and abilities. We find him as an expert in diagnosing human illnesses and as the veterinarian responsible for the bulls in the temple stables. He was the only person who could distinguish the living hypostasis of the god Apis and who was qualified to certify the purity of the animals to be sacrificed.

Examining a variety of sources, this essay will bring to light different functions and abilities of this officiant and characterize his double role.

Functions and abilities

As a doctor

Illness could be considered as a manifestation of the dangerous goddess' power that the *wab*-priest, by dint of his purity, could assuage and cure. Sekhmet's fury caused the illness; appeasing her cured it.

On another limestone statue of the *wab*-priest Iuny (Figure 1), we read that his father, Amenhotep, was not only head of the pure priests of Sekhmet, but also a chief physician. Graffiti on the walls of Amenhotep's chapel show that the tomb was a place of pilgrimage in the Ramesside period, probably attracting visitors who sought the intercession of Iuny and his father to heal ailments.

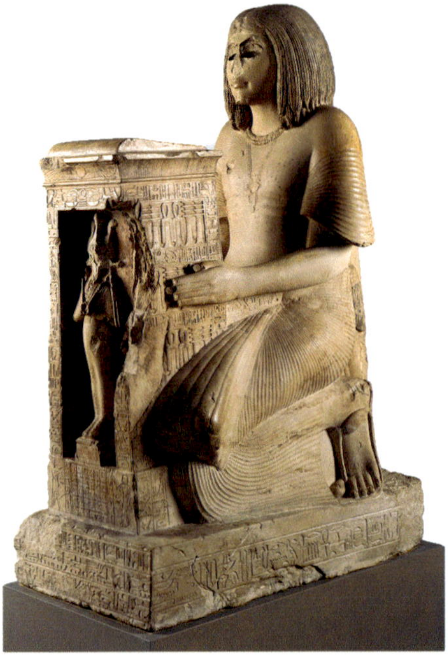

Figure 1. Kneeling statue of Iuny holding a shrine with a figure of the god Osiris, 19th Dynasty, Metropolitan Museum of New York, MET 33.2.1.

On an 18th Dynasty stela of another *wab*-priest called Nefer we read that he was a doctor (*swnw*) with skilful fingers, who had prescriptions with various applications and who had auscultated (*ḏ*ʿ*r*) the diseases of the body (Känel, 1984: 29-31).[2]

Thanks to their medical knowledge, *wab*-priests were also required to accompany members of mining and trading expeditions. In a hieratic graffiti from the early Middle Kingdom found in the alabaster quarries of Hatnub we find two personages, Herishefnakht (on the right) and Ahanakht. The former bears the titles of head of the priests of Sekhmet, head of the magicians and chief of the royal doctors, whilst the latter has only the title of priest of Sekhmet. Nevertheless, the texts that accompany each personage are practically identical. They are parallel versions showing that both practiced medicine. Both declared their skill in the diagnosis of illnesses:

Herishefnakht: 'Je suis directeur des prêtres-ôuab de Sekhmet, directeur des magiciens, chef des médecins du roi (...) Celui qui met sa main sur l'homme (malade) et qui le connait (son mal), celui qui est expert (dans l'art de) diagnostiquer avec la main...'.

Ahanakht: 'Je suis prêtre-ôuab de Sekhmet, expert en ses devoirs; qui met sa main sur l'homme (malade) et qui le connaît (son mal); qui est expert (dans l'art de) diagnostiquer avec la main; celui qui connaît les taureaux...'.[3]

Wab-priests are documented in the Edwin Smith and Ebers medical papyruses as specialists in the diagnosis of illnesses, along with other practitioners, such as the *swnw* and the *s*ꜣ*-srḳt*. In particular, we find them acting in the case of a scalp contusion laceration penetrating to the bone in the Edwin Smith papyrus [§1, col 1/2-12]. The text includes a remarkable explanation of the diagnostic process, defining it as a quantifiable science comparable to that of measuring and tabulating grain. It also contains a rudimentary explanation of the circulatory system, noting its origins in the heart.

By touching the patients, the *wab*-priests examined their blood circulation and diagnosed associated problems. The pulse was sequentially studied on the head, the hands, the *st-ib* and

[2] This stela was first published by Edwards, 1965.
[3] Hatnub, 15, 3-11. Transl. Känel (1984: 18).

the legs. Measuring or assessing the pulse gave them a direct indication of the condition of the patient's heart and their state of health. This is why the *wab*-priest Nefer is categorised as 'a true *swnw*, skilled with his fingers' in his autobiography engraved on the aforementioned stela.

As a propagator of illnesses

The *wab*-priests of Sekhmet presented a double characteristic: they propagated illnesses and cured them, a duality also found in the goddess they served. In the same way as the miasmas were transported on the breath of Sekhmet, the breath of the *wab*-priests was believed to be equally dangerous. Attested in Ebers Papyrus §855, the breath of a *wab*-priest in action could enter through the left eye and exit through the navel, causing terrible effects on the body:

> *ỉr ꜣḳ-ỉb mht-ỉb in ṯꜣw n rꜣ-ꜥ ẖry-ḥb ỉrr st*
>
> 'As for the forgetfulness of the heart (i.e. memory loss), it is the breath of the mouth (i.e. spell) of a lector priest that causes it' [PEbers 102, 4-5]
>
> *ỉr dḥrt nbt (…) ṯꜣw pw n rꜣ-ꜥ wꜥb*
>
> 'As for all bitterness (...) it is the breath of the mouth (i.e. spell) of a *wab*-priest.' [PEbers 100, 19]

This is due to the fact that once the goddess had been appeased and neutralised, Sekhmet's attributes were transferred to and assimilated by her officiant. This particularity of the *wab*-priests of Sekhmet could even be used to threaten the life of the Pharaoh, a fact that is exemplified in the delicate case of the 'conspiracy of the harem' in the reign of Ramses III.

The head of the pure priests of Sekhmet, Iyry, accused of casting spells against the Pharaoh, was forced to commit suicide, as is related in a passage of the so-called *Judicial Papyrus of Turin*, V, 4-5 (Känel 1984: 60-61). The magical procedures used in the attempted murder of the king are known from three more documents that form part of the so-called 'harem conspiracy dossier': the Rollin, Lee and Rifaud papyruses. From the Rollin papyrus we know the conspirators used potions to render human limbs powerless (Koenig 2001: 311). The medical knowledge of Sekhmet's pure priests could have been the reason why Iyry took part in the conspiracy by preparing those potions.

By chance, we know of the priest Iyry from other documents from Qantir, to the north-east of Bubastis. Interestingly, one of them is from the lintel of the door of his house, where we see him worshipping the names on the cartouche of Ramses III. The accompanying inscription tells us that that Iyry was also a king's scribe and a lector-priest. On a stela dedicated to Osiris, erected by his son, also a pure priest of Sekhmet, Iyry's name has been chiselled off, a *damnatio memoriae* probably due to his participation in the harem conspiracy (Habachi and Ghalioungui 1971: 67, Fig. 1-4).

As a doctor-veterinarian

Another of the functions of the pure priest of Sekhmet was to care for the stables of bulls. He was responsible for the herds of bulls of a temple, probably as a doctor-veterinarian. In some cases, we see that the *wab*-priests bore the title *mr iḥw* 'director of the bulls'. Although this is not a specific title of the *wab*-priest, it is interesting to note that *nbt iḥwt* 'lady of the bulls' is an epithet of the goddess Sekhmet in the litany of 360 names in the temple of Dendara (Känel 1984: 264).

A Ramesside ostracon from the 20th Dynasty found at Thebes bears the text of a letter in which the *wab*-priest Minmose is giving the *wab*-priest Sobekhotep certain recommendations on how to ensure the success of the posthumous worship of Amenhotep III (Känel 1984: 67).

Along the same lines, we find the following inscription in the south wall of the pronaos of Petosiris' tomb at Tuna el-Gebel. The daughters of this high priest of Thot pay homage to him, and one of them evokes the benefits the gods granted him during his life:

> 'Your herds are numerous in the stable, thanks to the science [lit. secrets] of the priest of Sekhmet.'[4]

On the hieratic graffiti in the alabaster quarries of Hatnub, mentioned earlier, the pure priest of Sekhmet, Ahanakht, is a *rḫ k3w* 'one who knows bulls', although this title may be more connected to proclaiming cattle as suitable for sacrifice than for healing ailing animals (Lord 2015: 146).

The god Apis was able to incarnate as a black bull and Sekhmet's priests had to ensure that the animal to be sacrificed did not bear any of the marks that identified it as the hypostasis of that god. Once examined and deemed suitable for sacrifice, the animal was marked on the haunches with a seal to avoid any confusion. In the Late Period, the seal was placed on the animal's horns (Känel 1984: 262). Herodotus tells us that if the animal had even a single black hair, it could not be sacrificed, as it was considered impure [Hdt. II 38].

According to Diodorus Siculus [1.85], once chosen, the young animal that would become the Apis bull remained in seclusion for forty days prior to its induction into the temple at Memphis. During this time women would perform the act of *anasyrmenê* before it to excite and hasten the calf's latent sexual powers (Morris 2007: 201). Similarly, the goddess Hathor exposed her private parts before Re-Horakhty in order to reactivate him, as his heart was very sore and he had fallen into a deep depression in the context of the long conflict between Horus and Seth [P. Chester Beatty I 3.10-4.3]. A small wooden automaton conserved in the Metropolitan Museum of New York [MMA 58.36] represents a naked goddess –with remains of Egyptian blue on her hair– covering her genitals with her right hand. When the string is pulled, the figurine raises her arm to reveal her genitals. This mechanical action eventually caused extensive erosion on the nose of the statuette, thus confirming it had been much used. Probably it was used during a temple rite re-enacting the episode of *The Contendings of Horus and Seth* related in the Papyrus Chester Beatty I.

In animal sacrifice

Another function of the *wab*-priest of Sekhmet was the control of the ritual slaughter of bulls[5]. Once the animal had been examined, a *wab*-priest of Sekhmet would have been present at

[4] Lefevbre 1924: 30, l. 16-17; Lord 2015: 146.

[5] Most of the evidence for this activity dates from the Old Kingdom and comes from scenes depicted in tombs and funerary temples. There are few scenes of bull sacrifice from the Middle Kingdom. In the New Kingdom there are

the moment it was slaughtered and butchered, in order to verify at first hand that the whole process had been carried out according to the rites. In Pathhotep's mastaba at Saqqara, the *wab* of Sekhmet, Unennefer, is witnessing a butchery scene (Känel 1984: 256). The pure priests inspected the entrails of the beast and its blood, smelling and perhaps tasting it, to see if it was pure and free of disease. This is why Irenakhti –a *mr wꜥb (Sḫmt) pr-ꜥꜣ swnw*– is depicted smelling the bloody hand of the butcher and proclaiming, 'it is pure!'. Känel (1984: 258-259) has demonstrated that Irenakhti was definitely a *wab*-Sekhmet priest. Examining the entrails and sniffing the blood of an animal are methods used in modern-day Egyptian villages to determine its health and edibility (Ikram 1995: 46).

In order to prevent spoilage of the meat, after the throat was cut the blood was drained from the body by pumping the foreleg, thereby forcing the blood to flow out (Ikram 1995: 46). The right foreleg (*ḫpš*), often represented as an offering to the gods, was considered the best piece of the animal, although more for religious rather than nutritional reasons. The foreleg was assimilated to Seth's arm, a weapon used to fight against enemies. In a fragment of a Ramesside stela in the Ny Carlsberg Glyptotek in Copenhagen there is a depiction of a bull-headed Seth facing Apophis in the bow of a boat. The inscription above qualifies him as 'bull of Ombos' (Figure 2). It is interesting to note that the hippopotamus, Seth's sacred animal, was called 'bull of the swamp', *kꜣ-mḥy* (Jasnow and Zauzich 2005: 343). Seth, characterized by his powerful front leg (*wsr ḫpš.f*), had his own sanctuary in the city of *Sper-meru* (in the nineteenth Upper Egyptian *sepat*), as mentioned in the Wilbour Papyrus: 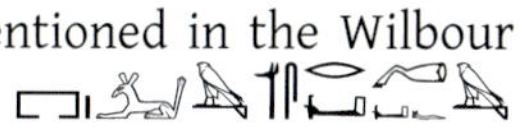 [Pap. Wilbour A 45, 11] (Torras 2016).

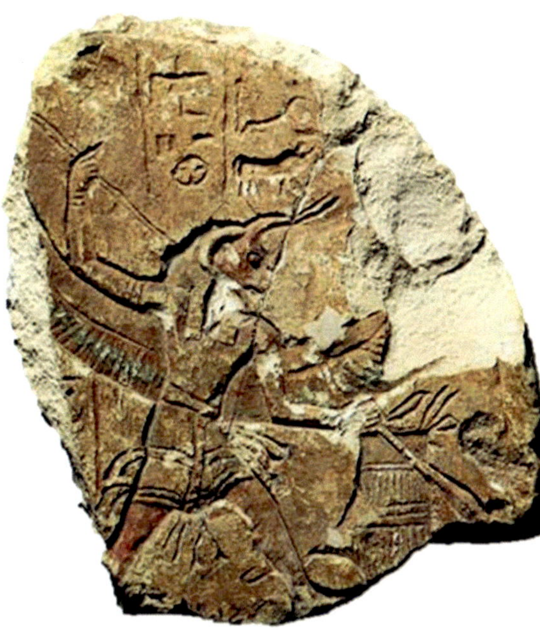

Figure 2. Upper right part of a round-topped limestone stela with a bull-headed, winged Seth in a barque spearing Apophis, 19th Dynasty, Ny Carlsberg Glyptotek (Copenhagen), ÆIN 726. Photo ©NCG.

In the nome-list incorporated into the so-called 'Vulture Text' in the Book of Thot, the name of the nineteenth Upper Egyptian nome is transcribed into Demotic script as *Wꜥbꜥb*.[6] Since the specialists have not yet agreed on a definitive reading of that region's name, this reference is particularly interesting, adding a new working hypothesis about the reading and meaning of this territory's name and emblem. This term read in Language of Tradition[7] can be translated as 'a pure one of horn' (*wꜥb-ꜥb*). This suggests us that it refers to the

more detailed scenes in temples, but without the *wab*-priest. In the 25th Dynasty we find copies of scenes from the Old Kingdom. Finally, in the Ptolemaic period the *wab*-priest is only mentioned in relation to this specific function in the temple of Edfu (Känel 1984: 265, n.1).

6 Papyrus Louvre E 10488, recto, L01 (V.T), x+2/18 (Jasnow and Zauzich 2005: 341, pl. 48).

7 The so-called *égyptien de tradition* was used for cultual and sacred geography texts such as the geographical processions engraved in late Egyptian temples (Torras 2016).

one who had been the main local god, Seth, but as a bull suitable for sacrifice. As mentioned above, in the Late Period the mark of purity consisted of a seal placed on the animal's horns. In addition, the Horus myth of Edfu explains that in this territory Horus cut the foreleg (*ḫpš*) of Seth [*Edfou* VI, 222, 2-5]. The Great Geographical Text of Edfu cites, as a local relic, 'the leg of the noble and Seth's testicles with the standard-holder below them': *sbḳw n sr is*(*wy*) *n Stš m i3t ẖr.sn* [Edfou I2, 342, 16]. In Greco-Roman texts, castration is normally mentioned in the context of animal sacrifice[8], meaning that the local relic in the nineteenth Upper Egyptian nome would have come from the castration of Seth in the form of a bull that was sacrificed. The local relic cited in the Great Geographical Text of Edfu offers a possible explanation for the region's emblem, composed of the hieroglyphic foot sign and two *was*-sceptres, 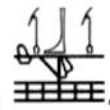.[9] We know that from the generalization of the outlawing of Seth's cult in the Late Period, the region's emblem underwent various theological reformulations designed to humiliate the god. It also had an impact on local cults and toponymy (Torras 2017b: 126-130).

In the Greco-Roman period, the *wab*-priest was called *moschosphragistēs*, 'the one who seals the calves' destined to be sacrificed. Two papyruses from second-century AD from El Fayum give the translation of the title in Demotic: *p3 wʿb Sḫmt*. Both texts are certificates of purity written in Greek with a Demotic subscription and refer to the same priest, Petosiris, who placed a seal on the bulls he had examined. From the seventh year of the Emperor Hadrian, it was decreed that all those who wished to sacrifice a bull had to present a certificate confirming the purity of the animal in which the *moschosphragistēs* had to indicate the number of animals examined and marked with a seal for each person (Känel 1984: 272-273).

Sacrificing a bull that had not been marked by a *wab*-priest was punishable by death or, according to other texts, with a strong pecuniary sanction and even ear and nose ablation. The type of sanction probably varied over time, becoming laxer in the Roman period (Känel 1984: 271).

Final remarks

The pure priest of the goddess Sekhmet was a type of ritualist closely linked to the Houses of Life. He had particular abilities for the protection of the country and the practice of medicine. He also played a veterinary role in ensuring the good condition of the bulls that lived in the temple stables.

Thanks to their purity they were able to assuage Sekhmet while being protected from the dangerous effects of the goddess' power. They were experts in the art of diagnosing illness by touching their patients, being 'skilled with their fingers'. However, the duality of Sekhmet –the furious one who kills/the satisfied one who vitalises– also characterised the priests who officiated at her worship. The spells and acts of Sekhmet's *wab*-priest could be considered the causes of disease and illness. In that respect, of particular significance is the participation of Iyry, a Sekhmet *wab*-priest, in the 'conspiracy of the harem' in the reign of Ramses III, rendering human limbs powerless.

[8] The Horus myth of Edfu reports the castration of Seth as a hippopotamus [*Edfou* VI, 75, 1-3]. Pap. Jumilhac III, 18-21; XX, 15-18 refers to the castration of Seth in the shape of a bull which is sacrificed (Te Velde 1967: 58, n. 8-59).

[9] According to another reformulation in the mythological Delta papyrus [pap. Brooklyn 47.218.84 XIII, 2-5], the toes of Sem, assimilated to Seth, were mutilated on the sacred mound of the nineteenth Upper Egyptian *sepat* (Meeks 2006: §32).

As we have seen, among the principal functions and abilities of the pure priests of Sekhmet was that of recognising the living hypostasis of the god Apis and of certifying the purity of the bulls to be sacrificed, as well as control of the death ritual of the bulls. The ritual slaughter and butchering of the bull under the supervision of this priest sought the prophylactic protection of Egypt.

Once the animal had been dismembered, the right foreleg (xpS) was assimilated to Seth's arm. This ambivalent god could be imagined as a bull-headed man fighting against Apophis and characterized by his powerful front leg in the nineteenth Upper Egyptian province. Although there he was the main local god, some arguments lead us to believe that, after his proscription in the Late Period, he was assimilated to the bulls suitable for sacrifice. From then on, this would offer an explanation for the region's name and emblem.

Finally, it is worth highlighting the survival of this officiant into the Roman period as a specialist in certifying the purity of the bulls to be sacrificed by a private individual. This shows the cultural resilience of ancient Egyptian traditions under Greco-Roman domination.

Abbreviations

Edfou I2 = Rochemonteix, M., E. Chassinat, S. Cauville and D. Devauchelle 1984. *Le temple d'Edfou*, t. I.2. *Deuxième édition revue et corrigé par S. Cauville et D. Devauchelle.* Cairo: Institut Français d'Archéologie Orientale.

Edfou VI = Chassinat, E. 1931. *Le temple d'Edfou*, vol. VI (Mémoires publiés par les membres de la Mission archéologique français au Caire 23). Cairo: Institut Français d'Archéologie Orientale.

Hatnub = Moeller, G. and R. Anthes 1964. *Die Felseinschriften von Hatnub.* Hildesheim: Georg Olms.

Hdt = Schrader, C. trad. 1977. Heródoto. Historia. Libro II, Euterpe (Biblioteca clásica Gredos 3). Madrid: Editorial Gredos.

P.Chester Beatty = Gardiner, A. H. 1931. *The Library of A. Chester Beatty: Description of a Hieratic Papyrus with a Mythological Story, Love Songs, and Other Miscellaneous Texts. The Chester Beatty Papyri, No. I.* London: Oxford University Press.

PEbers = Wreszinski, W. 1913. *Der Papyrus Ebers. Umschrift, Übersetzung und Kommentar I. Teil: Umschrift.* Leipzig: J.C. Hinrichs'sche Buchhandlung.

Urk. II = Sethe, K. 1904. *Hieroglyphische Urkunden der griechisch-römischen Zeit I. Historisch-biographische Urkunden aus den Zeiten der Makedonischen Könige und der beiden ersten Ptolemaër* (Urkunden des ägyptischen Altertums II). Leipzig: J. C. Hinrichs'sche Buchhandlung.

Pap. Wilbour = Gardiner, A.H. 1941. *The Wilbour papyrus. I. Plates.* Oxford: Oxford University Press.

Bibliography

Edwards, I. E. S. 1965. Lord Dufferin's Excavations at Deir El-Baḥri and the Clandeboye Collection. *The Journal of Egyptian Archaeology* 51: 16-28.

Habachi, L. and P. Ghalioungui 1971. The 'House of life' of Bubastis. *Chronique d'Égypte* 46/91: 59-71.

Ikram, S. 1995. *Choice Cuts: Meat Production in Ancient Egypt* (Orientalia Lovaniensia Analecta 69). Leuven: Peeters.

Jasnow, R. and K.T. Zauzich 2005. *The Ancient Egyptian Book of Thoth. A Demotic Discours on Knowledge and Pendant to the Classical Hermetica*, vol. 1: *Text*, vol. 2 : *Plates.* Wiesbaden: Harrassowitz.

Känel, F. von 1984. *Les prêtres- ouâb de Sekhmet et les conjurateurs de Serket* (Bibliothèque de l'École des Hautes Études 87). Paris: Presses universitaires de France.

Koenig, Y. 2001. À propos de la conspiration du harem. *Bulletin de l'Institut Français d'Archéologie Orientale* 101: 293-314.

Lefevbre, G. 1924. *Le Tombeau de Petosiris*, vol. II: *Les textes*. Cairo: Institut Français d'Archéologie Orientale.

Lord, C. 2015. One and the same? An investigation into the connection between veterinary and medical practice in ancient Egypt, in C. Price, R. Forshaw, A. Chamberlain and P. Nicholson (eds.) *Mummies, magic and medicine in ancient Egypt. Multidisciplinary essays for Rosalie David*: 140-154. Manchester: Manchester University Press.

Meeks, D. 2006. Mythes et légendes du Delta d'après le papyrus Brooklyn 47.218.84 (Mémoires publiés par les membres de l'Institut français d'archéologie orientale125), Cairo: Institut Français d'Archéologie Orientale.

Morris, E. F. 2007. Sacred and Obscene Laughter in *The Contendings of Horus and Seth*, in Egyptian Inversions of Everyday Life, and in the Context of Cultic Competition, in Th. Schneider and K. Szpakowska (eds.) *Egyptian Sotries. A British Egyptological Tribute to Alna B. Lloyd on the Occasion of His Retirement* (Alter Orient und Altes Testament 347): 197-224. Münster : Ugarit.

Te Velde, H., 1967. *Seth, God of Confusion. A study of his role in Egyptian myhtology and religion* (Probleme der Ägyptologie VI). Leiden: E. J. Brill.

Torras Benezet, N. 2016. *La sepat dels dos ceptres-uas a la llum de les processons geogràfiques: recerques en Geografia sagrada i 'teologia' local a l'antic Egipte.* Barcelona: PhD dissertation Universitat Pompeu Fabra - Institut d'Història Jaume Vicens Vives, http://www.tdx.cat/handle/10803/378044.

Torras Benezet, N. 2017a. Funciones y habilidades del sacerdote puro de Sekhmet: Rituales mágicos en el context del templo, in E. Suárez, M. Blanco, E. Chronopoulou and I. Canzobre (eds.) *Magikè Téchne. Formación y consideración social del mago en el Mundo Antiguo*: 15-31. Madrid: Dykinson.

Torras Benezet, N. 2017b. La província de los dos cetros-*uas*, un estudio de geografía cultual del antiguo Egipto. *Treballs de la societat catalana de geografia* 84: 115-132.

Yoyotte, J. 1980. Une monumentale litania de granit. Les Sekhmet d'Amenophis III et la conjuration permanente de la Déesse dangereuse. *Bulletin de la Société française d'Égyptologie* 87-88: 46-75.

A Historical Case. Dermatoglyphic Identification of Fingerprints of the TT 11 Tomb of Djehuty Project (1069 BC to 945 BC)

Berta Torrents Pérez
berta.torrents.perez@gmail.com
Podiatry, University of Barcelona

Pablo Martínez-Escauriaza Peral, Patricia Rodríguez Corbera
Podiatry, University of Barcelona

Rosa Dinarès Solà,
Autonomous University of Barcelona

Jesús Herrerín López
Autonomous University of Madrid

Abstract: Introduction: Fingerprints are visible characteristics that can endure invariably throughout an individual's lifetime, and sometimes even longer. This investigation analyses the fingerprints of four mummy digits found in Egypt, dating from *c.*3000 years ago. **Objectives**: The purpose of this study is to delimit the anatomical region where the samples belong to, to estimate its gender from the fingerprints ridge density, to establish the methodological lines in order to describe the samples and to determine and analyze the localized relationship between the frequency of minutiae and descriptive and anatomical variables with a main pattern. **Material and methods**: Only four of the 20 digits were recognized by the Automated Fingerprint Identification System (AFIS). The analysis of these four samples is accomplished through the lateral inversion of the finger pads with the AFIS. **Results**: We are dealing with four mummified digits from the old city of Thebes dated from the XXI-XXII dynasties of ancient Egypt, with feminine values regarding the gender determination. The main pattern that predominates is the loop ('*presilla*') and the fingerprints present a higher detectable number of minutiae than the current standard numeric value for forensic identification (ten-twelve characteristic points). **Discussion and Conclusions**: Therefore, it has been possible to establish the minutiae of the mummified fingers after 3000 years through a modern system such as the AFIS and with a result that would allow us to conduct a real identification; which highlights the exclusivity of this historical case.

Keywords: Fingerprints, Dermatoglyphs, Forensic Anthropology, Mummies.

Introduction

Fingerprints have been used extensively to establish human identity since 1890. This extensive use is due to the fact that no two people have the same impressions, not even monozygotic twins (Taduran *et al.*, 2016).

This study is part of the Djehuty Project, which I joined as a further member of the investigation through Dr Pablo Martínez-Escauriaza, Board of Directors of The American Society of Forensic Podiatry and member of the Djehuty Project, coordinated by CSIC and the *Ministerio de Economía, Industria y Competitividad* and *Ministerio de Educación, Cultura y Deporte del Gobierno de España*; in cooperation with Dr Jesús Herrerín, professor at the *Universidad Autónoma de Madrid* at the Department of Biology and Physical Anthropology; and Dra Rosa Dinarès, a forensic radiologist from the *Hospital Universitari General de Catalunya*.

Pharmacy and Medicine in Ancient Egypt
(Archaeopress 2021): 125–140

This study goes back to ancient Egypt, where identity and hierarchy were already of high social interest. The power that the Pharaoh possessed, together with the divine relationship that was granted to him, was such that only they and other influential people could commission their mummification (Samiento, 2010).

Djehuty project

The purpose of the Djehuty Project is the excavation, restoration, scientific publication and dissemination of a set of funerary monuments and burials of middle and upper class individuals, located on the Mount of Dra Abu el-Naga, at the northern end of the necropolis of the ancient city of Thebes, present-day Luxor, Egypt (Figure 1). The spotlight falls on the tombs of Djehuty and Hery, senior officials in the service of the royal administration around the year 1500 BC (Djehuty Project, 2018).

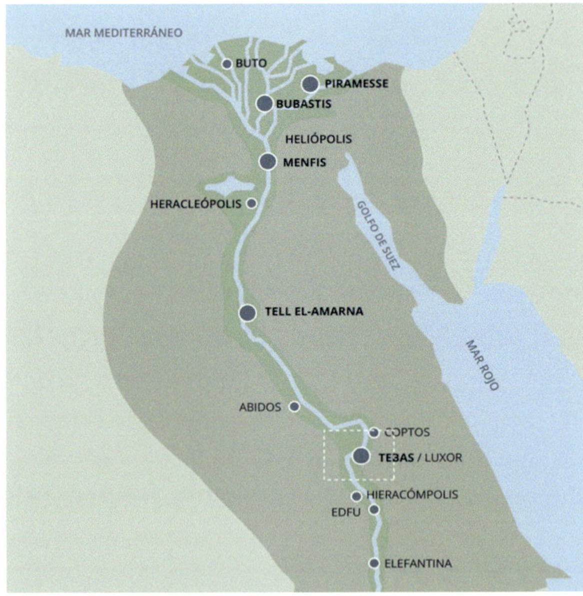

Figure 1. Localization of the Djehuty Project at Luxor, Egypt. Proyecto Djehuty 2018, *Excavación en Egipto*, viewed 8 May 2018, <http://www.excavacionegipto.com/index.php>

Djehuty TT 11 Tomb

The tomb of Djehuty was excavated in the south zone of the rocky hill of Dra Abu el-Naga, next to the grave of Hery. Both were discovered by J.F. Champollion at the beginning of the 19th century (AD 1829).

Djehuty was a supervisor of the priests of Hermopolis and later Overseer of the Treasury and of Works. He lived during the reign of Hatshepsut and Tutmosis III, around 1500 BC (XVIII dynasty) and he was an important personage at the time, with great influence within the government of Hatshepsut. In his autobiography he defined himself as a leader of the palace.

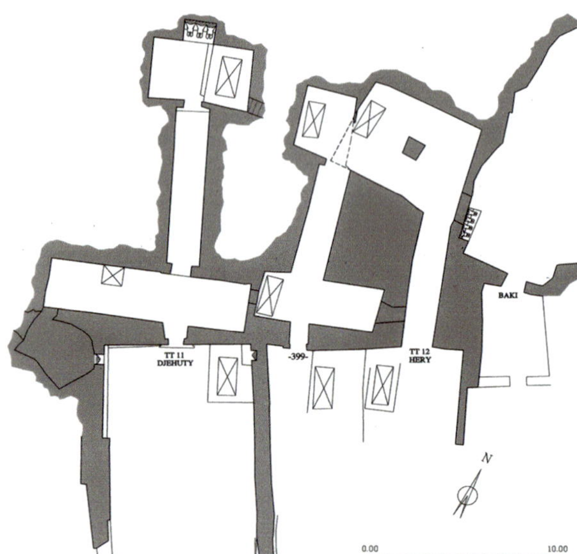

Figure 2. Map of the TT 11 Tomb of Djehuty. Proyecto Djehuty 2018, *Excavación en Egipto*, viewed 8 May 2018, <http://www.excavacionegipto.com/index.php>

Originally the tomb had an open entrance hall (Figure 2) without a roof, with a funeral panel, a statue of Djehuty and inscriptions on the walls with his biography. The first room (transverse room) contains tapestries of a banquet and funeral texts, along with stories of Djehuty with his father. This room leads to the main, long and narrow corridor, with reliefs of the river pilgrimage to Abydos (where the main temple of Osiris, king of the dead, is located) and ends at the entrance of the chapel, where engravings of funeral rituals and three statues of Djehuty with his father and his mother are located (Djehuty Project, 2018).

Mummification

During the XXI and XXII dynasties there were many political changes, the Pharaoh lost power and consequently an increase in robberies occurred in tombs of kings and nobles. This provided an opportunity for embalmers to see and restore mummies from earlier periods and, therefore, to learn about ancient mummification techniques. Consequently, they began to make changes in their techniques by bringing the technique of mummification to its most advanced point.

Each member and limb were bandaged separately, a careful internal mummification was conducted, and the bodies were dried with natron and often filled with resins.

Additionally, cosmetic treatments were applied to the mummies, with special attention to the nails which were tied with ropes. False eyes made of painted linen, glass or stone were placed in the mummies, which conferred a vivid appearance on them. The embalmers also treated the hair carefully, and mummies wearing wigs or extensions are often found.

Fingerprints

The impressions produced by the finger pads on inert surfaces, forming pictorial patterns, are known as fingerprints (Silva *et al.*, 2018). They have been described as immutable, perennial, varied and original; that is to say that each individual has individual designs, unique, and therefore different from those of any other human being. Three kinds of fingerprints can be differentiated (Martínez-Escauriaza Peral, Herrerín López and Gutiérrez-Redomero, 2017):

- Natural fingerprints: those that a person owns from before being born until after death.
- Artificial fingerprints: those that are obtained after inking and printing them in a postcard or dactyloscopic file.
- Latent fingerprints: those that are left impregnated in a smooth surface or in the skin.

The structures that produce these impressions are the dermatoglyphs, called dactylograms when referring to the fingerprints (distal phalanges). They are constituted by the ridges, papillary grooves and sweaty pores of the skin surface involving the epidermis and the dermis. They can be seen on the palmar aspect of the fingers, palms of the hands and feet, and they are specialized in the prehensile, locomotive and perceptive function of tactile stimuli (Silva *et al.*, 2018). Some syndromes have been described to cause changes in these digital designs, such as Basan syndrome, a rare syndrome with a dominant autosomal hereditary pattern that is characterized by a total absence of dermatoglyphs, among other signs (Blacker and LeBoit, 1993).

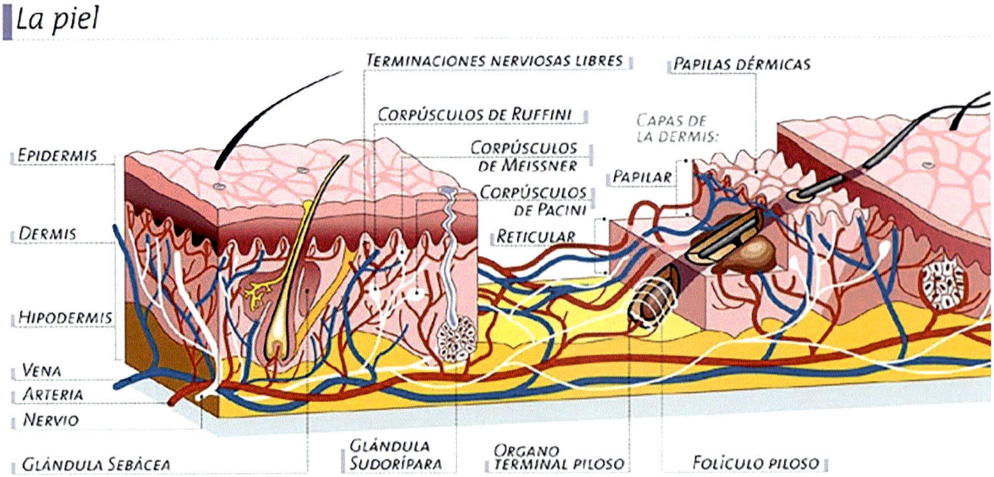

Figure 3. Anatomical structure of the skin. Martínez-Escauriaza Peral P, Herrerín López J and Gutiérrez-Redomero E 2017, 'Huellas dactilares, 3000 años después', *IX Jornadas de la Asociación Española de Antropología y Odontología Forense (AEAOF)* y IX *Reunión de la Sociedad de Odontoestomatólogos Forenses Iberoamericanos (SOFIA)*, La Rábida, Huelva, pp. 21.

Papillary ridges

They are an extension of what we know as dermal papilla, discovered in 1665 by Marcelo Malpighi, whose main function is to maintain the epidermis together. They are present in the friction areas of the skin of hands and feet and are located in the external papillary layer of the dermis (*FIGURE 3*), from where they originate unrepeatable forms that extend until emerging on the surface forming the papillary ridges (Martínez-Escauriaza Peral *et al.*, 2013).

Dactyloscopy

Dactyloscopy is the study of fingerprints and its origin dates back to 1892 thanks to Sir Francis Galton's publication of his pioneering work. This science has been widely used for human identification ever since (Lakshmi Kumari, Vijaya Babu and Kumar, 2014).

The most commonly used dactyloscopic system is the Vucetich, which describes four groups of main patterns in a fingerprint: arch ('*arco*'), whorl ('*verticilo*'), ulnar loop ('*presilla externa*') with a delta towards its left, or radial loop ('*presilla interna*') with a delta to its right (Figure 4). However, in order to classify and identify a digital fingerprint, it is necessary to resort to the so-called minutiae, the various forms presenting the papillary ridges (Gutiérrez Chávez, 2007), described in Annex I.

Types of dactyloscopic capacitation levels

In order to unify the international technical language when performing the analysis of fingerprints, a level classification is used (Martínez-Escauriaza Peral, Herrerín López and Gutiérrez-Redomero, 2017):

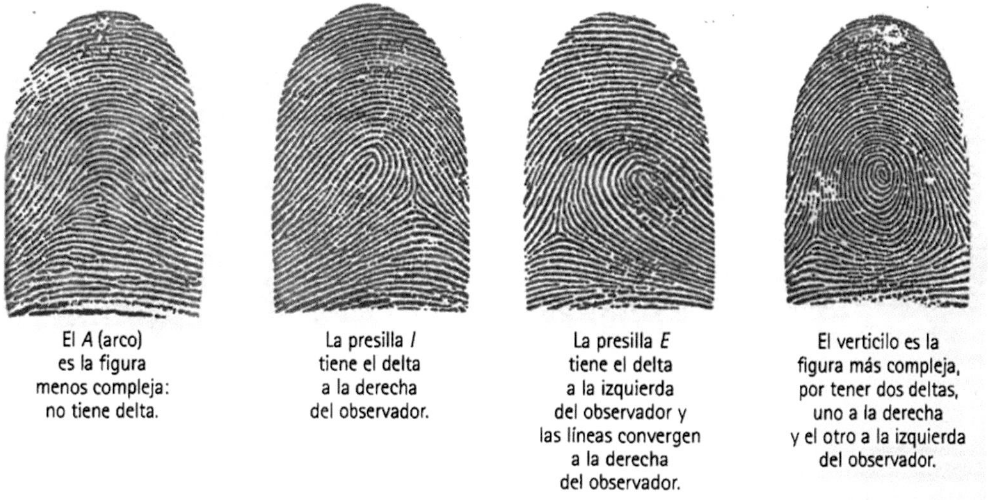

Figure 4. Types of main patterns in a fingerprint, from left to right: arch (structure without delta), radial loop (structure with a delta to the right), ulnar loop (structure with a delta towards the left), whorl (structure with double delta, one to the right and one to the left). Gutiérrez Chávez, A 2007, *Manual de ciencias forenses y criminalística*, 2nd edn, Trillas, México.

- Level I: the identification of the patterns of fingerprints, according to the ten-print classification system used by each country.
- Level II: the macroscopic analysis of the peculiarities of the papillary ridges, in order to verify the identity of the human being through their minutiae.
- Level III: the microscopic analysis of the peculiarities of the papillary ridges and the dimensions of the grooves, not visible to the human eye, to establish their biological originality and to corroborate the minutiae of Level II through poroscopy.

Forensic podiatry

Forensic science is used for the purposes of the law, particularly in the detection of crime and the administration of justice (DiMaggio and Vernon, 2017). Forensic podiatry is one of its medical subdisciplines, centered on human identification using the knowledge and experience of the podiatrist with a legal purpose (De la Cruz Pérez, 2017). That is to say, that together with forensic pathology, they are responsible for the examination of human bodies in order to determine the cause and the manner of death in criminal or suspicious circumstances, including the use of fingerprints for identification purposes (DiMaggio and Vernon, 2017).

HYPOTHESIS

- The realization of a necropapiloscopic analysis in the hydration of the fingerprints would determine the discrimination between genders of the subject/s.
- The identification of mitochondrial DNA and study with Carbon-14 would disclose the specific age of these individuals.
- The frequency determination of minutiae and the main pattern type of the fingerprints would allow us to perform an individual identification of the subject/s.

OBJECTIVES

1. To delimit the anatomical region to which the samples belong.
2. To estimate the gender from the density of the papillary ridges.
3. To establish the methodological lines for the description of the samples.
4. To determine and analyze the relationship between frequencies of minutiae and the descriptive and anatomical variables with a main pattern.

FINER CRITERIA

1. Feasible: This type of study is much more economical than a genetic analysis study of DNA or Carbon-14.
2. Interesting: These are digits that, despite their antiquity, preserve the dactylograms in a very good condition.
3. Novel: It is a historical case with which we had not come across, nor been able to study until now.
4. Ethical: It foments the identification of unknown people in the postmortem period - PM discriminating it with the dermatoglyphic reading of people in an antemortem period - AM.
5. Relevant: In the framework of forensic research, it underpins a scientific basis that verifies the current situation of lophoscopy.

Materials and methods

Materials

The sample of this study are fragmentary remains, digits pertaining to mummies of the XXI-XXII dynasty found in the well EU 165 of the tomb of Djehuty, excavated during the 2016 campaign of the Djehuty Project. The well, dated from the XVII dynasty, has a depth of 5.40 meters and leads to a funerary chamber at its western extremity.

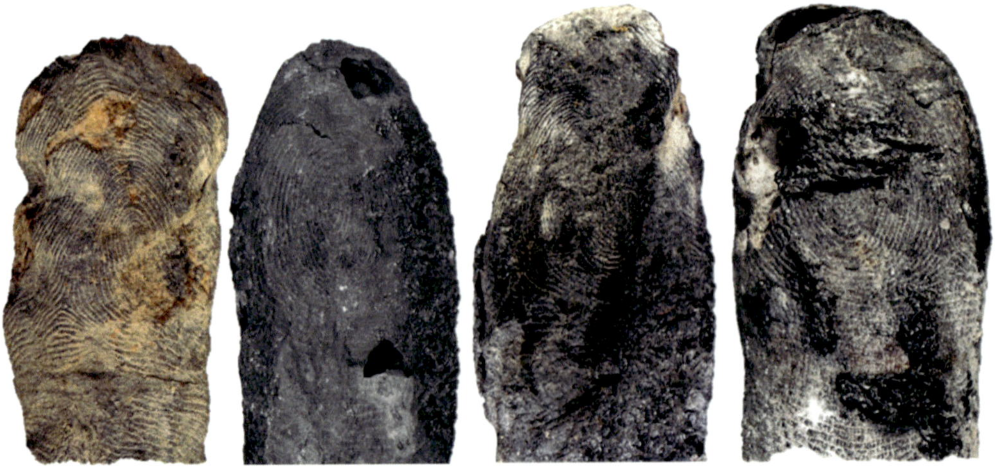

Figure 5. The four digits recognized by the AFIS. Assigned images by the Djehuty Project TT 11 team.

The elaboration and size of the chamber, larger than most, suggest that the tomb belonged to an important individual from the end of the 17th or early 18th dynasty. The tomb was reused during the XXI and XXII dynasties for probably six individuals. It was sacked violently, the coffins were broken in pieces and their mummies dismembered and scattered throughout the room (Djehuty Project, 2018).

Of the total of 20 samples obtained from the Djehuty Project, the ones that were not recognized by the Automatic Fingerprint Identification System (AFIS) were excluded. This left a total of 4 digits remaining (Figure 5).

Methods

The procedure for analyzing the obtained samples was as follows:

1. The 20 fingers found were photographed with metric references.
2. The fingers in which the dermatoglyphs were most significant and may be of greater analytical interest were selected.
3. The 20 fingerprints that were previously laterally inverted by being photographed directly from the finger pads through the AFIS were entered into the scanner.
4. A manual examination and analysis of the minutiae study was carried out, having been laterally inverted when being photographed directly from the finger pads.

By joining the study, the team of the Djehuty Project has provided me with the images and the necessary data to be able to develop the present work.

Additionally, a bibliographic search has been done in the Medline databases through Pubmed, Scopus and Google Academic, along with some book queries. The websites of *Diccionari Enciclopèdic de Medicina*, *Diccionari de l'Institut d'Estudis Catalans* and *Termcat*: center of terminology, have also been utilized for the correct use and translation of terminology and technical terms employed in this study. Due to the fact that the references of the technical words used for national security - in regards to minutiae and main fingerprint patterns - have been obtained from the *Cuerpo Nacional de Policía de España* and, therefore, written in Spanish, it was desirable to respect the reference language by accompanying the terms in question with the original word within brackets, and not translated.

Results

The four samples are identified as four digits from mummies dating from the XXI-XXII dynasty of ancient Egypt, obtained from the Tomb of Djehuty in Thebes, Luxor, during the 2016 campaign of the Djehuty Project. The four digits preserve their dactylograms with enough quality to be studied.

Regarding the estimation of gender, while waiting to be able to use other methodologies, we have obtained clear female values in the distal areas and values near the cut-off point in the proximal areas, although still within the female interval, by taking into account the density of ridges by defined area and using the correction factor on dehydrated tissues (15%) (Martínez-Escauriaza Peral, Herrerín López and Gutiérrez-Redomero, 2017).

The methodological lines established are the following (Figure 6):

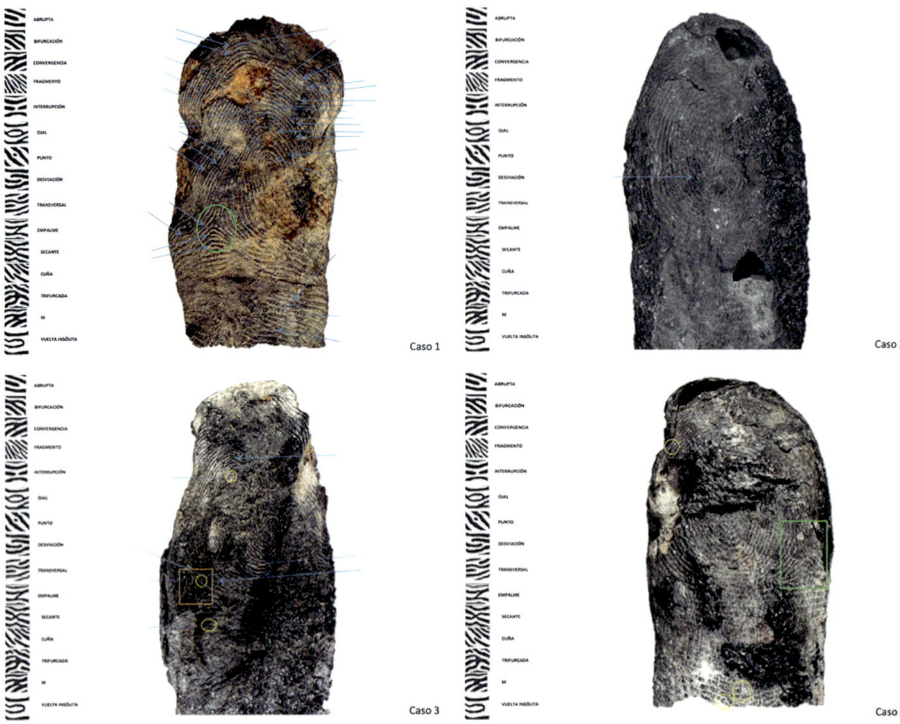

Figure 6. Results of the analysis with the AFIS. Assigned images by the Djehuty Project TT 11 team.

- The red color refers to the minutiae that appears as full coincidence between both fingerprints: the one introduced, in this case the mummy's, with the one that the system recognizes as a candidate. These points are found on both fingerprints in locations that the system considers similar.
- The yellow color corresponds to the points that the system has not identified in another candidate fingerprint, but that recognizes them as minutiae in the mummy's fingerprint.
- The other colors are the minutiae that the operator enters manually.

We have identified the frequency of appearance of the different types of main patterns: arch ('*arco*'), whorl ('*verticilo*') and loop ('*presilla*').

The most observed main pattern was the whorl (three of four), followed by the loop (one of four), and no digits have been identified with the arch pattern.

In both cases where it has been possible to identify the type of delta, a lateral open delta has been distinguished.

The number of minutiae found on the surface of the fingers, valued by the AFIS, exceeds the numerical standard in force in our country for forensic identifications (ten-twelve minutiae).

Discussion

It is important to emphasize that fingerprints of this age present the dactylograms and its corresponding minutiae so clearly, and that it has even been possible to analyze enough minutiae to allow the realization of a supposed identification (10-12 minutiae in Spain). All of this was achieved by laterally inverting the fingerprints when being photographed directly from the finger pads, therefore allowing its reading in a current system such as the AFIS after many years. It should be taken into account that despite the efficiency of computerized systems the manual expert's report will almost always provide more information and frequential appearance of minutiae than an analysis through the AFIS.

Due to the mummification and dissection process with natron, and the age of the corpse(s), there has been a general retraction of the tissues. This retraction affects the process of determining gender through the density of the papillary ridges since this is altered. Based on the correction factor on dehydrated tissues (15%) (Martínez-Escauriaza Peral, Herrerín López and Gutiérrez-Redomero, 2017) we were able to obtain results in spite of the retraction, feminine values in this case. In order to be able to ratify these results, a study of the genetic profile of mitochondrial and nuclear DNA of the samples could be carried out. However, that resource is more expensive and less accessible than the analysis of the papillary ridges of the digits.

The negative match results obtained with the AFIS (that there is no individual on the AFIS register whose fingerprints could be matched with those of the studied sample) are totally expected, since the ACE-V protocol (Analysis, Comparison, Evaluation and Verification) (Otero Soriano, 2012) was applied. In this process, the studied fingerprint is compared with the actual register of individuals from 21st century. Therefore, a positive match result would not be possible.

In reference to the ancestral pattern of the analyzed mummies, the possibility that the geographic area in which they were found is not their place of origin must be considered. Consequently, the analysis results of the minutiae or main patterns appearance frequency cannot be extrapolated at a geographical level of the area. It would be necessary to carry out a DNA study to be able to locate the individuals and determine their origin.

In this case, it has been difficult to transport and export the samples for the investigation in order to study them. It reflects a clear lack of unification of criteria in the international agreements between countries that would be suitable for facilitating the movement of these samples and favoring their study and analysis at a multidisciplinary and international level.

The use of the dactylograms is widespread in scientific research due to their characteristics of perpetuity, immutability, individuality and variety; its scope goes far beyond human identification. There are studies that claim that they can help determine the age of that fingerprint or even the blood group of an individual (Popa, Potorac and Preda, 2010) as well as their gender from the printed dactylograms (Taduran *et al.*, 2016; Eshak *et al.*, 2013; Tandon *et al.*, 2017) or pelmatograms (designs printed by the dermatoglyphs of the foot sole) (Kanchan *et al.*, 2012), for instance, at the scene of a crime, thus allowing the delimitation of a smaller group of suspects. They are also being used at a national security level to learn to distinguish a postmortem fingerprint from an ante-mortem fingerprint (Martínez-Escauriaza Peral *et al.*,

2013), especially to defend the identity and individuality of people and avoid criminal fraud through the use of fingerprints of deceased in official documents.

Forensic sciences also use skin annexes for the individualization, analysis and evaluation of samples. For example, the study of the nail matrix by conducting a toxicological analysis (additional or complementary to a capillary, venous and pilose analysis) to be able to know the drugs, medications or poisons that that individual consumed in the last months (Baumgartner, 2014; Krumbiegel *et al.*, 2016; Kuwayama *et al.*, 2017). Toenails are preferred when conducting these types of toxicological studies due to the slower growth they experience (30-50% slower than fingernails) and also because they are less exposed to environmental pollution. Therefore, they can provide information up to the last 14 months, whereas fingernails can only provide information up to the last 5 months (Baumgartner, 2014).

Dactyloscopy is used and studied in the same way outside the criminal field, for instance in sports as an indicator of personal athletic performance (Del Vecchio and Gonçalves, 2010), or in the medical field for the correlation it has with certain diseases such as asthma (Sun *et al.*, 2017), hypertension (Wijerathne *et al.*, 2015), caries (Asif, Babu and Naheeda, 2017), autism (Kazemi, Fayyazi-Bordbar and Mahdavi-Shahri, 2017; Stosljević and Adamović, 2013; de Bruin *et al.*, 2014) or arterial coronary pathologies (Lu *et al.*, 2015). It has correlation with some types of cancer too, such as intestinal cancers (Abbasi and Rasouli, 2017) or gynecological cancers (Abbasi and Rasouli, 2018), and also with some syndromes such as Downs Syndrome (Wojtowicz and Wajs, 2013; Asen, 2018), Naegeli-Franceschetti-Jadassohnde Syndrome (Tlish *et al.*, 2018) or Turner Syndrome (Jiménez-Madrid and Indira-Roncancio, 2018) as well as with the effect of certain antineoplastic drugs such as Paclitaxel (Azadeh *et al.*, 2017).

Studies have also been performed to correlate dermatoglyphs with innate intelligence, owing to the fact that they are formed during the same period in embryonic development as the cerebral neocortex (between the 13th and 19th prenatal weeks). The study of Lakshmi Kumari, Vijaya Babu and Kumar (2014) is based on the principle of multiple intelligence and on the fact that in individuals with intellectual disabilities there is an alteration or a common pattern on the fingerprints. They explain how in previous studies it has been shown that each digit is connected to a brain lobe and, therefore, related to a specific type of intelligence and a type of learning.

Currently, most studies support the properties of dermatoglyphs: their perpetuity, immutability, variety and individuality; excluding those cases in which the individual suffers from an illness that alters the design of the fingerprint or has undergone any alteration during the corresponding period of the embryonic development (for instance, the case of Thalidomide intake by the mother during pregnancy) (Lakshmi Kumari, Vijaya Babu and Kumar, 2014). Nevertheless, recent studies affirm that other factors such as senility can alter the perpetuity and immutability attributed to fingerprints (Silva *et al.*, 2018).

CONCLUSIONS

1. The obtained samples used in the study are four mummified fingers taken from the tomb of Djehuty, in the city of Thebes, belonging to the XXI-XXII dynasty of ancient Egypt.
2. It has been possible to determine the gender from the ridge density despite the retraction of the tissues and soft parts after so many years.

3. It has been possible to establish the minutiae after 3000 years of antiquity through a modern system such as the AFIS, obtaining a positive match, despite the fact that it is obviously not possible to recognize the identity of a human corpse from the 9th century BC in regard to a living person from the 21st century AD.
4. By means of the AFIS, it has been possible to determine the papillary ridges of the fingerprints of the mummified digits and their minutiae, conserved during the last 3000 years and presenting sufficient minutiae to conduct a supposed identification.
   The frequency values obtained in each fingerprint are characteristic of each subject and, therefore, unique and of a personal descriptive value of the individual to which the sample corresponds.

Bibliography

Abbasi, S and Rasouli, M 2017, 'Association between gastrointestinal cancers and fingerprint patterns in the Iranian population', *Genetics and Molecular Research*, vol. 16, no. 3.

Abbasi, S and Rasouli, M 2018, 'Dermatoglyphic patterns on fingers and gynecological cancers', *European Journal of Obstetrics & Gynecology and Reproductive Biology*, vol. 222, pp. 39-44.

Asen, D 2018, 'Secrets in fingerprints: Clinical ambitions and uncertainty in dermatoglyphics', *Canadian Medical Association Journal*, vol. 190, no. 19, pp. E597-E599.

Asif, SM, Babu, DB and Naheeda, S 2017, 'Utility of Dermatoglyphic Pattern in Prediction of Caries in Children of Telangana Region, India', *The Journal of Contemporary Dental Practice*, vol. 18, no. 6, pp. 490-496.

Azadeh, P, Dashti-Khavidaki, S, Joybari, AY, Sarbaz, S, Jafari, A, Yaseri, M, *et al.* 2017, 'Fingerprint changes among cancer patients treated with paclitaxel', *Journal of Cancer Research and Clinical Oncology*, vol. 143, no. 4, pp. 693-701.

Baumgartner, MR 2014, 'Nails: an adequate alternative matrix in forensic toxicology for drug analysis?', *Bioanalysis*, vol. 6, no. 17, pp. 2189-2191.

Blacker, KL and LeBoit, PE 1993, 'Congenital absence of dermatoglyphs', *Journal of the American Academy of Dermatology*, vol. 29, pp. 355–358.

de Bruin, EI, Graham, JH, Louwerse, A and Huizink, AC 2014, 'Mild dermatoglyphic deviations in adolescents with autism spectrum disorders and average intellectual abilities as compared to typically developing boys', *Autism Research and Treatment*, vol. 2014, pp. 1-6.

De la Cruz Pérez, A 2017, 'Clasificación pelmatoscópica de la región morfoanatómica plantar para la identificación humana: Metodología por impresión de solución yodada', Unpublished FDP (Final Degree Project), University of Barcelona, Barcelona.

del Vecchio, FB and Gonçalves, A 2010, 'Dermatoglifos como indicadores biológicos del rendimiento deportivo', *Revista Andaluza de Medicina del Deporte*, vol. 3, no. 4, pp. 38-46.

DiMaggio, JA and Vernon, W 2017, *Forensic Podiatry: principles and methods*, 2nd edn, CRC Press, New York.

Eshak, GA, Zaher, JF, Hasan, EI and El-Azeem Ewis, AA 2013, 'Sex identification from fingertip features in Egyptian population', *Journal of Forensic and Legal Medicine*, vol. 20, no. 1, pp. 46-50.

Gutiérrez Chávez, A 2007, *Manual de ciencias forenses y criminalística*, 2nd edn, Trillas, México.

Jiménez-Madrid, JH and Indira-Roncancio, T 2018, 'Mixoploid turner syndrome with a Y-chromosome structural aberration and its correlation with dermatoglyphs', *Ginecología y Obstetricia de México*, vol. 86, no. 2, pp. 137-145.

Kanchan, T, Krishan, K, Aparna, KR and Shyamsunder, S 2012, 'Footprint ridge density: A new attribute for sexual dimorphism', *HOMO - Journal of Comparative Human Biology*, vol. 63, no. 6, pp. 468-480.

Kazemi, M, Fayyazi-Bordbar, MR and Mahdavi-Shahri, N 2017, 'Comparative Dermatoglyphic Study between Autistic Patients and Normal People in Iran', *Iranian Journal of Medical Sciences*, vol. 42, no. 4, pp. 392-396.

Krumbiegel, F, Hastedt, M, Westendorf, L, Niebel, A, Methling, M, Parr, MK, *et al.* 2016, 'The use of nails as an alternative matrix for the long-term detection of previous drug intake: validation of sensitive UHPLC-MS/MS methods for the quantification of 76 substances and comparison of analytical results for drugs in nail and hair samples', *Forensic Science, Medicine, and Pathology*, vol. 12, no. 4, pp. 416-434.

Kuwayama, K, Miyaguchi, H, Iwata, YT, Kanamori, T, Tsujikawa, K, Yamamuro, T, *et al.* 2017, 'Time-course measurements of drug concentrations in hair and toenails after single administrations of pharmaceutical products', *Drug Testing and Analysis*, vol. 9, no. 4, pp. 571-577.

Lakshmi Kumari, K, Vijaya Babu, PVSS and Kumar, SV 2014 'Dermatoglyphics and Its Relation to Intelligence Levels of Young Students', *International Organization of Scientific Research - Journal of Dental and Medical Sciences*, vol. 13, no. 5, pp. 1-3.

Lu, H, Qian, W, Geng, Z, Sheng, Y, Yu, H, Ma, Z, *et al.* 2015, 'Dermatoglyphs in coronary artery disease among Ningxia population of North China', *Journal of Clinical and Diagnostic Research*, vol. 9, no. 12, pp. AC01-AC04.

Martínez-Escauriaza Peral P, Bartolomé Marqués R and Caballero D, Alfonso S 2013, 'Impresiones lofoscópicas postmortem', *Revista Española de Podología*, vol. 24, pp. 164-169.

Martínez-Escauriaza Peral P, Herrerín López J and Gutiérrez-Redomero E 2017, 'Huellas dactilares, 3000 años después', *IX Jornadas de la Asociación Española de Antropología y Odontología Forense (AEAOF)* y *IX Reunión de la Sociedad de Odontoestomatólogos Forenses Iberoamericanos (SOFIA)*, La Rábida, Huelva, pp. 21.

Otero Soriano, JM 2012, 'Policía Científica: 100 Años de Ciencia al Servicio de la Justicia', *Catálogo de Publicaciones de la Administración General del Estado*, Ministerio del Interior, Madrid, pp. 350.

Popa, G, Potorac, R and Preda, N 2010, 'Method for fingerprints age determination', *Romanian Journal of Legal Medicine*, vol. 18, no. 2, pp. 149-154.

Proyecto Djehuty 2018, *Excavación en Egipto*, viewed 8 May 2018, <http://www.excavacionegipto.com/index.php>.

Sarmiento, MM 2010, 'La construcción de la identidad del rey y los orígenes de su identificación con Osiris', *Trabajos y Comunicaciones*, pp. 293–309.

Silva, J, Rojas, M, Araya, C and Barraza, N 2018, 'Loss of the Dactylogram During Senility', *International Journal of Morphology*, vol. 36, pp. 258–261.

Stosljević, M and Adamović, M 2013, 'Dermatoglyphic characteristics of digito-palmar complex in autistic boys in serbia', *Vojnosanitetski Pregled*, vol. 70, no. 4, pp. 386-390.

Sun, L, Xue, W, Li, J, Zhou, Z and Han, W 2017, 'Palm dermatoglyphs and interleukin-4 receptor polymorphisms in asthma', *Biomedical Reports*, vol. 6, no. 1, pp. 21-26.

Taduran, RJO, Tadeo, AKV, Escalona, NAC and Townsend, GC 2016, 'Sex determination from fingerprint ridge density and white line counts in Filipinos', *HOMO - Journal of Comparative Human Biology*, vol. 67, pp. 163–171.

Tandon, A, Srivastava, A, Jaiswal, R, Patidar, M and Khare, A 2017, 'Estimation of gender using cheiloscopy and dermatoglyphics', *National Journal of Maxillofacial Surgery*, vol. 8, no. 2, pp. 102-105.

Tlish, MM, Sycheva, NL, Shavilova, ME and Psavok, FA 2018, 'Naegeli-Franceschetti-Jadassohn syndrome: A clinical-morphological diagnostic algorithm', *Voprosy Prakticheskoi Pediatrii*, vol. 13, no. 1, pp. 54-58.

Wijerathne, BTB, Meier, RJ, Agampodi, TC and Agampodi, SB 2015, 'Dermatoglyphics in hypertension: a review', *Journal of Physiological Anthropology*, vol. 34, pp. 29.
Wojtowicz, H and Wajs, W 2013, 'Classification of plantar dermatoglyphic patterns for the diagnosis of Down's syndrome', *Lecture Notes in Computer Science (including subseries Lecture Notes in Artificial Intelligence and Lecture Notes in Bioinformatics)*, vol. 7803, no. 2, pp. 295-304.

Acknowlegements

I would like to thank Dr Pablo Martínez-Escauriaza and Patricia Rodriguez for their support, guidance and motivation throughout the creation of this study and Dra Rosa Dinarès, Dr Jesús Herrerín and the rest of the Djehuty Project for letting me be part of the research team and giving me this extraordinary opportunity.

Annex

Annex I. Morphology and abbreviations of minutiae

TABLE 1. Morphology and abbreviations of minutiae. *Cuerpo Nacional de Policía, Gobierno de España.*

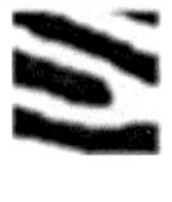	A	**RIDGE ENDING ('*Abrupta*'):** Papillary ridge that being confined among other two ridges of greater length is interrupted definitively. They are classified in two types: initial (when starting from the left side of the dactylogram the ridge begins) and final (when starting from the left side of the dactylogram the ridge is interrupted).
	B	**BIFURCATION ('*Bifurcación*'):** Point in which a papillary ridge that starts from the left side of the fingerprint is split into two ridges.
	C	**CONVERGENCE ('*Convergencia*'):** Point in which two papillary ridges that start from the left side of the fingerprint are merged into one.
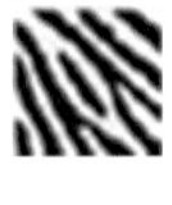	F	**INDEPENDENT RIDGE or FRAGMENT ('*Fragmento*'):** Ridge with both 'ridge ending' ends and variable length: 'small' if the length of the fragment is less than five times the width of the ridge, and 'large' if the length of the fragment is five to ten times greater than the width of the ridge.
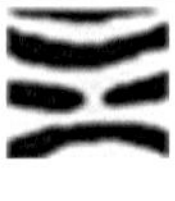	I	**BREAK ('*Interrupción*'):** A space that shortens the trajectory of a complete ridge, as long as it is not greater than twice the width of the ridge, nor less than the width of the ridge. The extremities that delimit the interruption must be rounded off.
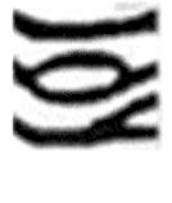	O	**LAKE or ENCLOSURE ('*Ojal*'):** A space more or less elliptical formed by the branches of a bifurcated ridge that re-merged by convergence. Depending on the length of the bumps, they can also be classified as large and small, following the same criteria set forth for the 'independent ridge'.
	P	**POINT or DOT ('*Punto*'):** Small ridge fragment, as short as wide, that is usually located in the middle of an interruption, in a united delta or between two ridges, being able to appear attached to any of these.
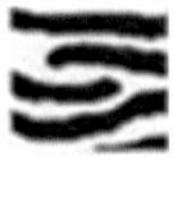	D	**OVERLAP ('*Desviación*'):** A point where two ridges from opposite sides do not find themselves, leaving them separated by an interpapillary groove (overlapping no more than triple the width of the ridge).
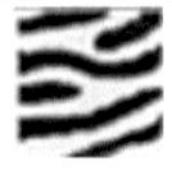	T	**CROSSBAR ('Transversal'):** Ridge that deviates from the main direction and crosses between two ridges of opposite direction.
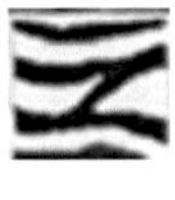	E	**BRIDGE ('Empalme'):** Short ridge of oblique or perpendicular direction that fuses by its ends with other two parallel ridges.
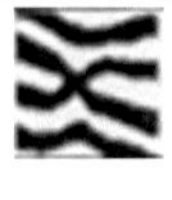	S	**CROSSOVER or OPPOSITED BIFURCATION ('Secante'):** Point of contact between two ridges that immediately separate, forming a blade.
	CU	**DOCK ('Cuña'):** Point formed by three 'ridge ending' ridges in which one of them enters, not more than three times the width of the ridge, at the beginning of the interpapillary groove formed by other two ridges that run in the opposite direction.

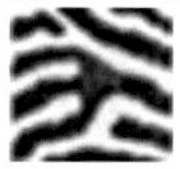	TF	**TRIFURCATION ('Trifurcación'):** Point from which a ridge branches into other three. They can be classified in two types: with a divergent direction (when starting from the left side of the dactylogram, the ridge is ramified in three) and with a convergent direction (when starting from the left side of the dactylogram, three ridges are merged into a single ridge).
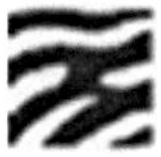	M	**M SHAPE ('En M'):** Point where two convergences and a bifurcation come together or vice versa. They can be classified in two types: with a divergent sense (when starting from the left side of the dactylogram we find first two bifurcations and then a convergence), and with a convergent sense (when starting from left side of the dactylogram we find first a bifurcation and then two convergences).
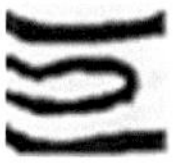	V.I.	**RETURN ('Vuelta Insólita'):** Ridge that abruptly changes its direction bending itself extending even in the opposite direction to the principal ridge, without getting to constitute a nuclear center, meaning that it is not seconded by the bordering ones. It can be simple or double.